Prevention
Across the Life Span:
Healthy People
For the Twenty-First Century

American Nurses Association
Council of Community Health Nursing

Edited by Ruth N. Knollmueller, Ph.D., R.N.

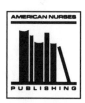

American Nurses Publishing
is the publishing program of
the American Nurses Foundation,
an affiliate organization of the
American Nurses Association.

This book was developed by the American Nurses Association's Council of Community Health Nursing.

ISBN 1-55810-091-1
Published by
American Nurses Publishing
600 Maryland Avenue, SW
Suite 100 West
Washington, DC 20024-2571
CH-27   5M   11/93

Table of Contents

Foreword

The next century will inaugurate a new millennium. We face a future so vast in its human dimension that it will "defy prediction while posing momentous questions about social and economic viability and human vitality in the face of a new era" (U.S. Public Health Service, *Healthy People 2000: National Health Promotion and Disease Prevention Objectives*).

The past century of biomedical research has taught us that health and a better quality of life are within each individual's grasp—from the pregnant woman to the older adult. Prevention is a key to open doors to improving health, avoiding disease, and developing the potential of individuals to achieve healthy life styles. Heart disease and cancer are the leading causes of death and can be prevented with the knowledge we have acquired in this century.

Prevention will be a major focus of health care initiatives for the next century. Many disciplines have attempted to publicize efforts in prevention. There are limited texts that address prevention on a holistic basis, though most deal with specific disease entities. This particular text addresses holistic prevention across the life span.

Nurses are poised in positions in health care to have a major impact on wellness, health promotion, and disease prevention. The belief that the health care system needs restructuring to guarantee access to care, contain costs, and ensure quality care will guide nurses in health care reform. As nursing attempts to build its foundation and realize its goals, a visionary plan is being developed to include essential health care services. Prevention and screening are among the core services envisioned. A major paradigm shift from illness and cure to wellness and care will provide the framework for services.

Because of the lack of a specific prevention publication addressing all age groups, the Council of Community Health Nursing of the American Nurses Association prepared this publication, *Prevention across the Life Span: Healthy People for the Twenty-First Century.* Our goal is to empower individuals to assume responsibility for health care and to challenge nurses to investigate the current research and develop futuristic programs.

Virginia Trotter Betts, J.D., M.S.N., R.N.
President
American Nurses Association
Washington, DC

Preface

Not long ago, I called the pediatrics department of the health maintenance organization (HMO) to which our family subscribes and inquired about whether our two teenage daughters might be considered for re-immunization for measles. I indicated that they had been given their initial measles, mumps, and rubella vaccinations at the age of twelve months, the recommended age at the time. I was informed that the measles vaccine was very costly and that there was no supply to cover re-immunizations. There was only enough to provide for those children who were currently eligible for this immunization and for those children defined as "at risk."

Although that reasoning seemed plausible at first, the more I thought about it, the more I felt that my HMO should, in fact, be contacting me about this question rather than the other way around. Further, there was an epidemic of measles in our area at the time, requiring schools to cancel their spring proms and other events drawing crowds because it was too complicated and difficult for the young people to prove their immunization status. Clinical complications from the disease were catching the interest of the newspapers as the state health department issued notices about the need for adequate immunization and the seriousness of a measles infection. One dramatic case described the tragic event of a young college-age student who became ill with measles (having been immunized according to the earlier schedule), was gravely ill in a hospital, and on life support with the expectation of permanent residual.

I began an extensive correspondence with the physician chief of the pediatrics department from whom I would receive a reply stating there still was no clarity about the efficacy of re-immunization from the American Academy of Pediatrics and other official sources, and emphasizing the cost of such a program for their eligible population of subscribers. I countered that prevention of the disease was the most cost-effective approach regardless of the immunization costs. The letters from the HMO were always polite but the decision was made; there was to be no re-immunization. In a desperate final attempt to capture the attention of our primary care providers, I then requested that a blood titer be done to determine that our daughters were adequately protected against measles since re-immunization was not a consideration. Soon after that request, I received a phone call indicating there was now enough vaccine available and that I could bring our daughters into the HMO to receive it. We went the same day!

This episode took place over a period of nearly a year. It is an example of how difficult it can become to secure an easily prescribed preventive intervention. The outcome was acceptable because of my sheer tenacity and the knowledge that I knew my request was an appropriate one.

It is disturbing, at the very least, to have a provider who publicly purports to place a value on prevention and health promotion but is not willing to practice it. Resistance to implementing prevention practices, either from individuals or organizations in our health care provider systems, may be driven by the initial cost. The denial of potential future costs incurred as a result of the absence of prevention, continues to govern the decisions of our policy makers and those who are in a position to allocate funds for the purpose of preventing illnesses and promoting good health practices.

This volume is dedicated to sharing information and supporting the practice of prevention and health promotion. There is important data in this book that demonstrate how we, as nurses in community health nursing, do truly affect the health status of the populations we serve. The hope of each of us who has contributed to this book is that we, and all of you who read it, will continue in our commitment toward *Prevention across the Life Span: Healthy People for the Twenty-First Century.*

Commentary
Prevention across the Life Span: Healthy People For the Twenty-First Century

Ada Sue Hinshaw, Ph.D., R.N., F.A.A.N.
Director
National Institute of Nursing Research
National Institutes of Health
Bethesda, MD

and

Janet Heinrich, Dr.P.H., R.N., F.A.A.N.
Executive Director
American Academy of Nursing

Prevention across the Life Span: Healthy People for the Twenty-First Century is timely from the perspective of a national research agenda and the national need for health care reform. Recent biological, behavioral, and sociocultural research has already influenced patterns of health care in the United States, with greater changes expected in the near future. A good example is our understanding of the human immunodeficiency virus (HIV) and the rapid scientific documentation of the factors related to the progression of related diseases and health behaviors. Just as we are blending the physical and biological sciences for a better understanding of the precise molecular detail of proteins and other biologically important molecules to develop vaccines and understand diseases, we need to blend the behavioral and social sciences to understand the role of behavioral factors in health and disease.

Several of this book's authors speak to the need for more prevention research. Dr. Simmons addresses the critical need for good data on the cost-effectiveness of prevention strategies as well as documentation of their clinical effectiveness. The need for better descriptive information on sociocultural factors related to health and illness and tested culturally sensitive interventions is clearly articulated by Dr. Spector. Dr. Williams's review of research in prevention helps link the research effort with the clinical and policy implications. Dr. Williams also provides a framework for future research directions with an emphasis on community interventions and community-wide studies.

The National Institute of Nursing Research (NINR), as a part of the National Institutes of Health (NIH), is committed to improving the health of the public through the support of research and research training. Although many of the institutes have active programs of research in the areas of disease prevention and prevention-related research that targets behaviors for specific diseases, NINR is concerned as well with understanding health promotion and the contextual factors that influence healthy life styles for all ages, groups, families, and communities.

Health promotion among children and adolescents is one of seven priority areas being developed by NINR. The paper by Dr. O'Sullivan outlines the issues during this developmental state that need further study if we are to find constructive ways of encouraging healthy choices. NINR is supporting a cluster of studies that address *low birth weight* (LBW). Culturally sensitive interventions to prevent LBW and pregnancy complications are being developed and tested with several diverse populations of high-risk women. Another project is examining the effects of culture on the prevalence and patterns of abuse during pregnancy, a topic described in Dr. McFarlane's chapter.

There is a tremendous need as well as tremendous opportunities for nurse scientists to be involved in community-wide interventions as defined by Dr. Williams. NINR is working with the Office of Disease Prevention at NIH and other funding agencies on a major Women's Health Initiative that will target community-wide prevention interventions. Schools, churches, and work sites are settings that several investigators are using to test health promotion strategies. NINR has also developed collaborative efforts with other funding agencies supporting community-based studies to add nursing interventions to existing protocols.

Several papers address the need for common measures of outcomes in order to compare findings across service settings and populations. There is also a need for research findings to undergird *Nursing's Agenda for Health Care Reform*, (ANA 1991). There is interest in testing existing models of care that provide essential services, including health promotion activities by nurses. It is also critical to develop and test new models of care such as the one described by Dr. Flynn in the Healthy Cities Indiana Project.

Prevention services are not available to all citizens of our country through current health insurance programs. Dr. Smith articulates the current public policy dilemmas in relation to individual responsibility for health and the social environments for health. She describes a health policy conceptual model that places health promotion clearly within a societal context. These social and cultural factors need to be understood better if we are to be successful in reaching our goal of a healthy nation.

Commentary
Prevention across the
Life Span: Healthy People
For the Twenty-First Century

Marla E. Salmon, Sc. D., R.N., F.A.A.N.
Director, Division of Nursing
Bureau of Health Professions, Health Resources and Services Administration
U.S. Department of Health and Human Services
Rockville, MD

This is a book about prevention. It was written for nurses and by nurses. Its purpose is to help nurses fulfill their potential as key providers of preventives services. There are three underlying premises in this book: 1) preventive services are of great benefit to people of all ages—from preconception to senescence; 2) nurses can play key roles as preventive services providers; and, 3) without adequate knowledge and skill, nurses will not play such a role.

How does this book enable nurses to overcome some barriers that often keep them from being key preventive services providers? These barriers, for the most part, are based on misconceptions or myths about nurses and nursing. Stating the myth, countering it with a different perspective, and referring the reader to sections of this book, will help the reader begin to see ways to become better equipped to practice *Prevention across the Life Span*.

Myth 1: All nurses are prepared to practice prevention. If prevention is understood as the movement of social, economic, political, environmental, biological, and medical forces to eliminate the possibility of a health problem occurring, then it simply is not true that all nurses are prepared to practice prevention. What is true is that nurses come with an orientation toward health and the total person. This orientation serves as an excellent foundation for building the specific knowledge and skills relating to primary intervention with respect to the many determinants of health mentioned above. In this book the reader will find excellent perspectives relating to sociocultural (Dr. Spector), economic (Dr. Simmons), sociopolitical determinants (Drs. Flynn and Smith) of health. These chapters provide insight into both the "state of the present" and ideas about where we need to go in these areas. Where we need to go as a profession in the area of prevention is discussed both in terms of its research implications (Dr. Williams) and the future for nursing (Dr. Knollmueller).

Myth 2: Once you have the basics, you can provide preventive services to anyone. Unfortunately, prevention is not at all like riding a bicycle. Prevention is more like shooting at a moving target. The word, target, is very important in this sense. Prevention, by definition, must be targeted. To provide effective preventive services, one must understand what one is trying to prevent and for whom. As such, one must know the nature of the problem to be prevented, the determinants of that problem (social, political, environmental, biological, economic, and so on), and effective interventions at both individual and macro levels. The categories of interventions remain largely the same: education, engineering, enforcement. How each of these is expressed for any specific problem varies. They also vary depending on level of intervention—e.g., whether individual, family, community. The chapters relating specifically to age groups or special populations all provide insight into the specific potential target problems and preventive approaches to these.

Myth 3: Nurses can be effective in preventive strategies without the assistance of others. Professional isolation or exclusivism is anathema to successful preventive efforts. By simply considering what determines health and illness, it is easy to see that these factors cross disciplines both within and outside health care. To be effective, nurses must identify those key disciplines and potential collaborators as part of planning and implementing interventions. The very nature of prevention is interdisciplinary. The challenge for nurses is to bring the best of nursing to the table in helping to orchestrate effective interventions, not to maintain separation. Drs. Flynn and Raines present a real-world case study of interdisciplinary, community-based collaboration. They also discuss the theory base for this important approach.

Myth 4: We have enough nurses to provide the care we will need in the future. There are many good reasons for prevention—the human, social, and economic benefits are tremendous. One additional important reason for prevention, however, is simply that unless we become better at preventing the need for complex secondary and tertiary care, including nursing care, we will continue to experience a worsening shortage of nurses over the next few decades. Based on how we currently utilize nurses, which is mostly in secondary and tertiary care settings, we will need to produce twice as many nurses each year as we do now simply to maintain a balance between supply and demand. It is highly unlikely that we will be able either to afford or to produce those numbers of nurses. We need to find better ways of utilizing nurses and assuring that they have an early and lasting impact on the health of the people they serve. In Dr. Knollmueller's chapter on the future of prevention, she proposes some important mechanisms for utilizing nurses better toward this end.

Myth 5: There are plenty of resources available for nurses to learn about prevention. Maybe. There are, in fact, increasing numbers and sources of information regarding the whole area of prevention. Much of it is found in the public health literature. What we continue to need in nursing are resources that help nurses effectively bridge the fields of nursing and public health and that are written with nurses in mind. This is not to say in any sense that those resources that are not nursing-specific are not relevant. Rather, it is very useful to have compendia, source books, and guides for nurses that help to ground them in the area of prevention. These can serve as foundations for further building with other specialized literature relating to prevention.

Myth 6: Once a nurse has the knowledge and skills, successful preventive strategies will take place. Yes and no. Knowledge and skills are clearly crucial components of preventive services. However, they don't assure that the services will be furnished. There are three other key ingredients, none easily taught. The first is leadership. The complexity of activities required to mount truly effective preventive strategies requires that someone "move" the forces necessary. In other words, prevention doesn't simply happen. Prevention is, by its very nature, cross-sectoral, interdisciplinary, and outside of any one person's job description. Because of the breadth of their preparation, nurses are often in a good position to provide that leadership.

The second prerequisite is creativity. Effective strategies require resourceful and creative approaches because there are seldom enough people or dollars available for comprehensive preventive services. Creativity, or the ability to find alternative approaches and engage the efforts of others (paid and voluntary), is critical to effective approaches. The third ingredient is courage. Prevention is, unfortunately, still overshadowed by the high-tech, tertiary-care–oriented nature of our health care system in the United States. For preventive services to become a part of every person's health services experience, health care providers will have to stand up and advocate such services in a variety of settings, including the political arena. As this country moves toward health care reform, the nature of that reform will be determined by those who have the most impact. Nurses oriented toward prevention will need to step forward, have the courage to be counted, and become part of the political reality of prevention.

This book should be viewed as a foundation for nurses as we move toward more and more preventive services in all of our roles. It serves to introduce the reader to a broad spectrum of understanding, knowledge, and next steps relating to nurses playing key roles in prevention.

The views expressed in this commentary are those of the author only and not necessarily those of the U.S. Department of Health and Human Services or the Health Resources and Services Administration.

Commentary
Prevention across the
Life Span: Healthy People
For the Twenty-First Century

O. Marie Henry, D.N.Sc., R.N., F.A.A.N.
Deputy Surgeon General, Public Health Service (retired),
U.S. Department of Health and Human Services

The chapters selected for this book address many vital components of the health promotion and prevention crusade. Several focus on prevention activities for specific population groups such as infants, children, adolescents, new mothers, adults, and the elderly. These chapters provide us with many new insights about ways to work with these groups. Other chapters contain provocative reviews of topics such as the economics of prevention, the development of community coalitions, sociocultural perspectives on prevention, current research issues relating to prevention, and health promotion as a public policy goal. These papers provide a framework for the direction nursing must take to implement nursing knowledge in the nation's movement toward the goal of a healthy America.

I believe that the emphasis which began in 1979—the new and strong emphasis on prevention and health promotion—was absolutely right. The evidence linking life style factors and health led to the conclusion emphasized in the 1979 Surgeon General's Report, *Healthy People,* i.e., that further improvements in the health of the American people would not be achieved by increased medical care but through a national commitment to prevent disease and promote health.

We must capitalize on these trends, both individually and collectively. Our society must face the fact that we have the individual capacity and responsibility personally to control the quality of our own health and well-being. Nurses can play a major role in mobilizing the health care system to advance the cause of prevention.

The art of balancing the technological imperatives with disease prevention is an exacting one. However, prevention should be the intervention of choice whenever and wherever possible. Prevention will help us to sustain and extend our lives, and teach us how to protect ourselves from disease and injury. The movement toward prevention across the life span has always been a part of the mission of public health nursing and is now beginning to spread to other health care professions. Prevention is also an important life style focus for an increasing number of people. However, if nursing is to play a major role in ensuring healthy people for the twenty-first century, we must be clear as to what role nursing can play in realistic, objective measures rather than in aspirational terms. We are in a position to make a true difference in the health of the American public through prevention.

After perusing these chapters, I am confident that you will be more enthusiastic than ever about the invaluable role that health promotion and disease prevention can play in eliminating or alleviating many of the costly, painful, and debilitating maladies that affect far too many of our fellow citizens.

Commentary
Prevention across the
Life Span: Healthy People
For the Twenty-First Century

Constance A. Holleran, M.S.N., R.N., F.A.A.N.
Executive Director
International Council of Nurses
Geneva, Switzerland

This book is being published by the American Nurses Association (ANA) at a most appropriate time. Prevention is a topic one hears discussed frequently these days. National and international news magazines have cover stories on vitamins and prevention of aging, and television features increasingly focus on wellness and how to maintain it.

Internationally, which is where my focus tends to be, there is an upsurge of interest in the environment, nutrition, and poverty as they relate to illness and stages of wellness. Various United Nations agencies are organizing conferences along those lines and the "Safe Motherhood" initiative is being funded by groups such as the World Health Organization (WHO), UNICEF, other United Nations agencies, the World Bank, and private foundations. Dr. McFarlane and Ms. Patwari graphically describe why this effort is so important.

Recently, the relationship of health status of a country to its level of economic development has being highlighted (we nurses recognized it long ago.). Dr. Simmons makes some very clear, concrete suggestions as to how nurses can increase their influence in health policy development in the prevention of illness. Dr. Spector emphasizes the need for cultural sensitivity in working with people from backgrounds different from our own—i.e., how we personally relate to the person (quietly or aggressively, eye contact or no eye contact, and so on) as well as to what we suggest and how we teach them.

Such sensitivity, much of which can be learned throughout a career, applies as well to working within any community. The coalitions organizing that Drs. Flynn and Rains refer to applies to our clinical work but also to our professional activities with colleagues in nursing, in other professions, and in universities. It is important to learn the skills of coalition-building and then to practice them regularly. This was one of the most important things I learned in my work in ANA's governmental affairs department in the 1970s. Such skills can make a tremendous difference in achieving one's set goals to improve the health status of various groups and a community as a whole.

Success in eradicating certain communicable diseases in some countries and decreasing their incidence in others is one of the major accomplishments of the health community worldwide. Though much remains to be done, the data show the encouraging progress being made.

Because neonatal tetanus, respiratory illnesses, and severe diarrheal diseases continue to plague children in much of the world, prevention efforts must be strengthened. Education of mothers to achieve literacy and improvement of sanitation, transportation, and nutrition are elements that we know have great influence on the prevention of childhood illnesses.

Judith Igoe identifies the more common childhood health problems encountered in the United States. Among them is one with which the developing world is becoming much too familiar: HIV infection. It is a problem for children directly as many are born HIV-positive. It is also a problem for whole communities which are experiencing a tremendous increase in the number of children who are orphans as a result of AIDS deaths, often of both parents. The economics of families, villages, cities, and whole countries are being affected by the loss of working-age people, with results only now beginning to show in parts of Africa, Asia, and North America.

International health and prevention programs have not yet adequately focused on children once they reach school age. It is a gap nurses need to fill. They need also to draw the attention of government and other providers to the needs of these children. Effective prevention efforts in childhood will save money in the long run.

Dr. O'Sullivan and Ms. Tesoro address the importance of adolescent health. Only four years ago, I was told by some leading nurses in developing countries that adolescent health programs are a "western" concept. They do not have them or need them. In reflecting on that I decided that in those countries one goes from childhood to adulthood very rapidly. This is evidenced by very early marriage and childbirth in the teen years. Happily, WHO recently added an adolescent health focus to its family health program.

Nursing's contribution and responsibility for prevention (and care) of chronic illness in all age groups is carefully described in the chapter by Drs. Macnee and Goeppinger. Strategies are suggested that can help us to think more carefully about ways to help people live comfortably and productively.

Mr. Fehir focuses our attention on several work-site prevention needs. At the International Council of Nurses (ICN), safety in the workplace and protection of workers' health (including that of nurses) has been a major activity. Currently, ICN is urging nurses worldwide to become better informed about substance abuse. This ties in to the United Nations Decade against Drug Abuse, which began in June 1992. Many nurses still need to get themselves better informed on this major health problem.

Dr. Kathleen Beckman Blomquist speaks to some of the quality-of-life factors that older people worldwide—not just in the United States— desire. Longer life spans and the migration of younger family members away from their families have caught some countries unprepared for the change in the roles of older family members. To have to rely on care by outsiders is something unusual for people in many cultures. This area is also one the ICN has been working on. The 1992 International Nurses' Day theme was "Healthy Aging," which focused on prevention of illness and disability. Our posters and educational kits obviously met a great need for information. So it is good to see that topic prominently addressed in this publication.

Dr. Carolyn Williams cites data that should make each of us pause to assess our efforts in prevention for every age group and for every practice location—schools, homes, workplaces, and health facilities. She suggests several research possibilities that need to be acted on soon.

The final chapter deals with my area of special interest, that of health policy. Drs. Smith and Wesley remind us that increasingly the public expects to take responsibility for maintaining its own health.

Dr. Knollmueller takes us into the future and discusses ways that the individual nurse can help achieve the agreed-to health goals for the year 2000. Such a premise is one of the foundations of the "Health for All by the Year 2000" (through primary health care) programs of WHO. Health education, proper nutrition, and sanitation are among its key elements.

To refocus the health expenditures of any country, constructive influence and leadership by nurses and nursing organizations must be even more effective. ANA has long led in this regard which, at ICN is one of our highest priorities.

Reading this book has once again made me aware of the universality of nursing and the issues it faces in all parts of the world.

1

The Economics of Prevention

Susan J. Simmons, Ph.D., R.N.
Senior Policy Analyst, Office on Women's Health, Public Health Service
U.S. Department of Health and Human Services
Washington, DC

It is a timeless axiom that an ounce of prevention is worth a pound of cure. What follows from this, however, is *not* that prevention is worthwhile simply because it saves money, but, instead, because it promotes health at a reasonable price. Mobilizing the creativity and commitment of the nation in the interest of prevention is now recognized as both a health and economic imperative.

Healthy People 2000: National Health Promotion and Disease Prevention Objectives (U.S. Public Health Service 1990) represents a challenge to achieve three major prevention goals: increase the span of healthy living, reduce health disparities, and achieve access to preventive services for all Americans. To meet these goals, 300 measurable objectives have been established under the categories of health promotion, health protection, and preventive services. Health promotion objectives refer to personal choices about life style behaviors, such as physical activity and fitness, nutrition, tobacco use, alcohol and other drug use, and family planning. Health protection objectives address environmental measures for ensuring the safety of large population groups. Preventive services objectives involve screening, immunization, and counseling interventions for individuals in clinical settings.

Although the beneficial effects of prevention on health are well known, the associated cost effects are not as clear. This chapter addresses economic factors that influence the delivery of preventive health care in the United States. The content of the chapter is organized into four sections: 1) clinical effectiveness of preventive health care; 2) cost-effectiveness of preventive health care; 3) current coverage policies for preventive health care; and, 4) strategies for enhancing the delivery of preventive health care. The discussion has been prepared by assembling comments in these areas from a variety of groups concerned with the economics of preventive health care, including federal government agencies, health insurance groups, and professional health organizations.

In this chapter, preventive health care is broadly defined as any interaction between a health care provider and a client that promotes health and prevents illness, disability, and premature death. More specifically, preventive health care consists of counseling, screening, and immunization services designed either to inhibit the occurrence of disease or injury (*primary prevention*) or to detect and treat risk factors for disease or injury (*secondary prevention*).

Clinical Effectiveness of Prevention

Establishing the impact of prevention on health has preceded establishing its impact on economics. The clinical effectiveness of prevention was validated with the publication of the U.S. Preventive Services Task Force report, *Guide to Clinical Preventive Services* (1989). The report provides age- gender-, and risk factor–specific recommendations for the prevention of more than sixty major causes of morbidity and mortality. The methodology of the report involved rigorously reviewing and grading the quality of scientific evidence regarding the effectiveness of three types of clinical preventive services: screening tests, immunizations, and counseling.

With an inherent understanding of the value of disease prevention and health promotion, nursing is uniquely positioned among health disciplines to benefit from the task force findings. Because nursing has long emphasized forging partnerships with clients in the interest of promoting and maintaining health, the task force report provides documented justification for nurses to assume leadership roles in preventive health care delivery. The data suggest that counseling interventions to change personal health behaviors of clients long before the onset of clinical disease are the most promising role for prevention in current health care practice. The report indicates that both providers and clients must assume responsibility for health maintenance, with the client being responsible for behavioral change.

Cost-Effectiveness of Prevention

The push for prevention to be judged according to whether the gains in health are a reasonable return for the costs incurred occurs at a time when the nation continues to be burdened economically by preventable illness, injury, and disability (see Table 1.1). The portion of the gross national product (GNP) going to health care expenditures rose from 5.3 percent in 1960 to over 11 percent by 1990, amounting to more than half a trillion dollars (Health Care Financing Administration 1990). The diagnosis and treatment of disease conditions—e.g., heart disease, cancer, injuries, and low birth weight—have outstripped society's ability to pay for what are essentially preventable conditions.

Understanding how financial resources are, and should be, used in preventive health care involves consideration of one of three models: *investment, insurance,* or *consumption* (Eisenberg 1988). In the investment model of prevention, today's cost is weighed against the financial

Table 1.1   Costs of Treatment for Selected Conditions

Condition	Overall magnitude	Avoidable intervention[1]	Cost per patient[2]
Heart Disease	• 500,000 deaths per year • 284,000 bypass surgeries per year	–Coronary bypass surgery	$ 30,000
Cancer	• 510,000 deaths per year • 1 million new cases per year	–Lung cancer treatment –Cervical cancer treatment	$ 30,000 $ 29,000
Injuries	• 142,500 deaths per year • 2.3 million hospitalizations per year • 177,000 spinal cord injuries	–Quadriplegia treatment/ rehabilitation –Severe head injury treatment/ rehabilitation	$570,000 (lifetime) $310,000
Alcoholism	• 105,000 alcohol-related deaths/year • 18.5 million people abuse alcohol	–Liver transplant	$250,000
Low birth weight babies	• 23,000 deaths/year • 260,000 low birth weight babies born/year	–Neonatal intensive care for low birth weight babies –Care for low birth weight babies	$ 10,000 $ 31,000
Inadequate immunization	• Lacking basic immunization series: –20 to 30 percent age 2 years or younger	–Congenital rubella syndrome treatment	$422,000 (lifetime)

*Source: *Healthy People 2000* p. 5. Data compiled and updated to June 1991 dollars from various sources by the Office of Disease Prevention and Health Promotion.
[1]Examples (other interventions may apply).
[2]Representative first-year costs, except as noted. Not indicated are non–health care costs, such as lost economic productivity.

consequences of tomorrow's event. Cost-effectiveness analysis has been the most popular method of approaching prevention as an investment decision. In essence, cost-effectiveness analysis measures the net cost of providing a service (expenditures minus savings) as well as the outcomes obtained. Expenditures include direct costs (e.g., screening tests, provider visits) and indirect costs (e.g., time spent exercising or attending health education class). Outcomes are reported either as a single clinical outcome (such as years of life saved) or as several outcomes combined on a common scale (such as quality-adjusted life years). The primary purpose of cost-effectiveness analysis is to help clinicians and policy makers focus on investments that bring the most health for the required expenditure.

Evaluation of prevention's cost-effectiveness has lagged behind evaluation of its clinical effectiveness. A number of fundamental questions remain about the cost-effectiveness of prevention, even when the services are of demonstrated clinical value. Providing coverage for preventive services is likely to increase costs, which is problematic in an era of escalating health care expenditures (Russell 1986). Furthermore, cost-effective preventive health care with established clinical value may lose its efficiency when performed by different providers employing different techniques. A special difficulty is encountered when determining the cost-effectiveness of counseling services, which are often open-ended and variable. In such cases, the methodological weaknesses of the analyses override most attempts at pricing such services.

Thus far, cost-effectiveness analyses of preventive services have included screening for lead, cholesterol, and cervical cancer for older low-income women, and mammography for women sixty-five years old and older. Each of these interventions indicates different costs per year of healthy life, suggesting that whether a preventive intervention is judged cost-effective should also depend on personal and social values. Although cost-effectiveness analyses provide essential information, they should not force choices. With the estimates of costs and health effects before them, clinicians, scientists, and policy makers must still ask themselves: Are these health effects worth the costs? According to Weinstein (1990), "The appropriate standard of comparison is not a positive economic profit, but a cost-effectiveness ratio comparable with or superior to those of other health care practices" (p. S89).

Insurance and consumption are two alternative models of economic decision making in prevention. The insurance model stipulates that spending in the present will avoid a potential adverse outcome in the future. Rather than seeking positive outcomes in the future, insurance decision makers attempt to avoid negative future outcomes (i.e., risk aversion). The insurance model typically involves incorporating pooled funds in anticipation of a low-probability event.

In contrast to investment or insurance, the consumption model considers prevention as an expenditure providing benefits today (for example, a sense of well-being from physical activity). Considering prevention as a good to be consumed today places the emphasis on active prevention: individuals expending the time, energy, and money to change behavior, with the possibility of an immediate payoff.

Whether prevention is viewed as investment, insurance, or consumption depends on which model best explains preventive behavior and services delivery. Although none of these three may fully explain prevention, when taken together they may assist in understanding how resources are, and should be, used for disease prevention and health promotion—the next topic for discussion.

Paying for Preventive Health Care

The U.S. health-care financing system has evolved with an historical bias toward financing the diagnosis and treatment of acute illnesses. Despite their demonstrated effectiveness, preventive services continue to be excluded from many public and private insurance plans, thus contributing to their under-utilization (Davis, Bialek, Parkinson, Smith, and Vellozzi 1990). Because of the variability in extent of coverage for preventive health care, it is important to distinguish between several types of payment systems.

Public Insurance

Medicare.   When it was established in 1965 as the federal program to finance health care for the elderly and disabled, Medicare was barred by statute from paying for preventive services. Since that time, however, a growing number of preventive services have been covered under Medicare, including pneumococcal vaccine; hepatitis B vaccine for those at high or intermediate risk; cervical cancer screening; and mammography. In addition, Medicare beneficiaries enrolled in HMOs are frequently covered for additional services, such as eye, ear, and dental examinations as well as health education services.

Medicaid.   As the federal/state government program that finances health care for certain groups of low-income individuals, Medicaid has covered a number of preventive services. Mandatory services are of two major types: family planning services; and *early/periodic screening, diagnosis*, and *treatment* (EPSDT) for those under 21 years of age. In addition to the mandatory services, a number of states provide other services as optional benefits—e.g., wellness checkups, fluoride treatment of teeth, immunizations, and genetic screening.

Recent legislative expansions of the Medicaid program now provide coverage to pregnant women and children in families with incomes between 133 percent and 185 percent of the federal poverty level. This broadened eligibility is intended to address infant/childhood morbidity and mortality, which are related to the lack of preventive health care coverage for these groups.

A core package of preventive health services for Medicare- and Medicaid-eligible adults has recently been drafted for internal review by the U.S. Department of Health and Human Services. This package, which is based on the recommendations of the U.S. Preventive Services Task Force (1989), provides a minimum set of age- and gender-specific benefits (i.e., risk assessment, immunizations, targeted physical exams, and risk-specific counseling) for inclusion in periodic health visits. It is estimated that this type of preventive health care can be provided at an average cost of $46 per person per year to a well population.

Private Insurance

Commercial insurance carriers have been reluctant to provide coverage for preventive health care. This is because health insurance plans were originally established to provide coverage for acute illnesses treated in hospital settings. Prevention has never been a principal component of health insurance policy.

In recent years, however, some companies have expanded coverage for preventive health care by creating optional packages to indemnity plans, at an added cost. Insurers are also increasingly covering preventive services as part of their managed care programs. In some cases, states have instituted coverage policies in which carriers are required to provide coverage for certain preventive services. For example, several states have recently enacted laws that require insurers to reimburse clients for routine mammograms.

A reflection of the gradual broadening of coverage for preventive health care is found in the screening guidelines issues jointly by the American College of Physicians and the Blue Cross/Blue Shield Association (BCBSA) in June 1991. BCBSA is now providing its customers with a model preventive services package, which includes screening tests for breast, colon, cervical, and lung cancer; heart disease; hypertension; diabetes; thyroid disease; and osteoporosis. BCBSA estimates the annual cost of insuring these adult screening services to be approximately $36 per individual or $90 per family. In the broader category of health promotion, a recent BCBSA survey indicates that 70 percent of BCBSA plans are either developing or marketing programs that include health education programs and healthy life style incentives.

Health Maintenance Organizations

In contrast to indemnity plans, HMOs, *preferred provider organizations* (PPOs), and other managed care plans are more likely to provide a broad range of preventive care services. Because HMOs offer comprehensive benefits to a large enrolled population for a fixed fee, there is an incentive to encourage preventive care that can reduce the need for costly treatment of illnesses. In addition to the minimum services required by federal law, such as well-child care, periodic health examinations, and voluntary family planning services, HMOs provide other services, such as health education about specific conditions and behavioral change programs. Although nearly half of all HMOs require co-payment, the fee is minimal, usually no more than $5 per visit.

Work Site Programs

In recent years, coverage for certain preventive services, such as well-child care and mammograms, has begun to appear in some employer plans, particularly as a result of collective bargaining for that service. Preventive services are also covered increasingly by employers through their managed care programs. In addition, many employers have begun offering screening tests in controlled environments, such as on-site or at a setting negotiated by the employer.

The National Survey of Worksite Health Activities, sponsored by the U.S. Department of Health and Human Services in 1985, found that nearly 66 percent of work sites with more than fifty employees provide at least one prevention program. The most frequently cited programs include smoking cessation, health risk appraisal, back care, stress management, exercise, and injury prevention. Most programs are funded by the company.

Enhancing Preventive Health Care Delivery

Given the importance of prevention in improving and maintaining the health of the public, it is critical for nursing to articulate an agenda that will ensure the delivery of effective preventive health care for all Americans. The beginnings of such an agenda are evident in the report *Nursing's Agenda for Health Care Reform* (ANA 1991), a broad-based strategy for restructuring the health care system. The report calls for a federally defined standard package of essential health care services, including preventive services. Also emphasized is the development of provider/client relationships, directed at prevention activities, that will ultimately improve health outcomes in a cost-effective manner.

The following recommendations serve as a multi-pronged strategy that addresses the economic and sociopolitical issues supporting an equitable preventive health-care delivery system in the United States.

1. Develop position papers on prevention policy issues. Manuscripts, monographs, and other formal presentations of viewpoints should be developed by nursing groups concerned with economic, practice, education, or research issues in prevention. One approach would be to evaluate the *Healthy People 2000* report and identify how organizational activities are supporting achievement of the Year 2000 objectives. In any event, it is important to link relevant policies and programs to the broader national prevention agenda. By doing so, nursing not only takes its place at the policy table but also is able to have a significant impact on prevention issues.

2. Provide testimony to expert groups. Clearly developed position papers on prevention must be presented before governmental bodies. Congressional committees, the Health Care Financing Administration (HCFA), insurance groups, employers, trade associations, the Physician Payment Review Commission (PPRC), and Congress' Office of Technology Assessment (OTA) are among the entities responsible for determining economic policy in prevention. These and other groups should be the recipients of high-quality, clear, and realistic testimony from nursing.

3. Influence consumer expectations about prevention. Delivering prevention talks to community organizations and information to the news media will help to raise public awareness of prevention and its value in promoting health. Efforts to influence consumer demand for preventive services likewise is valuable in promoting coverage of such services.

4. Demonstrate the cost-effectiveness of prevention. More data are needed concerning prevention's cost-effectiveness relative to its clinical effectiveness. Establishing a comprehensive database for cost-effectiveness research is a necessary first step. Using common measures of outcome is required in order to compare findings across services and populations. Well-conducted economic evaluations and literature reviews should be helpful in convincing Congress, employers, and insurers to expand coverage for preventive services.

5. Improve reimbursement for preventive health care. Increasing consumer demand for preventive care, and provider willingness to offer such care, are substantial forces in favor of the coverage of preventive services in health insurance plans. Several methods of payment have been suggested, including fee-for-service, which remains the dominant method of payment for health care services.

Nursing should continue to lobby for equitable reimbursement according to the resource-based relative value scale. A potentially preferable approach may be to establish a periodic preventive-health visit fee, which would specify a package of preventive services for different population groups. In this case, payment would be conditional upon providing all services within the package, although not all services would need to be provided during a single visit.

Nursing should participate in a broad range of activities that evaluate options for expanding coverage of preventive health care. HCFA is currently sponsoring a series of demonstration projects concerned with cost-effectiveness issues and alternative methods of payment for preventive services. Opportunities for nurses include serving on grant review panels evaluating economic issues in prevention, or being members of project teams that are collecting or analyzing cost-effectiveness data. For proposals seeking to expand reimbursement for preventive health care to be acceptable politically, research such as that being conducted by HCFA and OTA should be carefully monitored by interested nursing groups. An ongoing reinforcement of coalitions with organizations concerned about preventive care is most important. With a combination of approaches, clinical effectiveness and cost-effectiveness of preventive health care can be further emphasized and the goals of health promotion and disease prevention realized.

References

Davis, K., Bialek, R., Parkinson, M., Smith, J., and Vellozzi. 1990. Paying for preventive care: Moving the debate forward. *American Journal of Preventive Medicine* 6(4, supplement), 7–30.
Eisenberg, J.M. 1988. Discussion of economic barriers to preventive services: Clinical obstacle or fiscal defense? In *Implementing preventive services*, eds. R.N. Battista and R.S. Lawrence, pp. 121–126. New York: Oxford University Press.
Health Care Financing Administration. 1990. National health expenditures, 1988. *Health Care Financing Review* 11(4), HCFA Pub. No. 003298.
American Nurses Association. *Nursing's Agenda for Health Care Reform.* 1991. The Association: Washington, DC.
Russell, L. 1986. *Is prevention better than cure?* Washington, DC: Brookings Institution.
U.S. Preventive Services Task Force. 1989. *Guide to clinical preventive services. An assessment of 169 interventions.* Baltimore: Williams & Wilkins..
U.S. Public Health Service. 1990. *Healthy people 2000: National health promotion and disease prevention objectives.* U.S. Government Printing Office: Washington, DC.
Weinstein, M.C. 1990. The costs of preventions. *Journal of General Internal Medicine* 4(6, supplement), S89-S98.

2

Sociocultural Perspective of Prevention

Rachel E. Spector, Ph.D., R.N., C.T.N.
Associate Professor
Boston College School of Nursing
Chestnut Hill, Massachusetts

Community health nurses are entering the 21st century dealing with enormous demographic, social, and cultural changes. Many of these play a dramatic role in consumers' preventive health care beliefs and practices and their use of community health nursing services. This chapter addresses the demographic changes occurring in this country and the sociocultural factors that serve as barriers to the use of preventive health care services, a phenomenon it behooves community health nurses to consider.

Demographic Change

One need only compare the 1990 and 1980 censuses to see how the people of our nation are changing. In 1980, the population of the United States was 226.5 million: 83.2 percent white, 11.7 percent African American, 0.6 percent Native American, 1.5 percent Asian/Pacific Islander, 3 percent other; that is, 16.8 percent were people of color (it should also be noted that 6.4 percent claimed Hispanic origin, but could be of any race). In 1990, despite an estimated headcount shortfall of 5.3 million people—many of whom were non-white and Hispanic city dwellers (Sege and Mashek 1991)—the overall population of the United States was 298.7 million: 80.3 percent white, 12.1 percent African-American, 0.8 percent Native American, 2.9 percent Asian/Pacific Islander, 3.9 percent other, or 19.7 percent people of color. In 1990, 9 percent of the population claimed Hispanic origin

11

but could be of any race (Barringer 1991). Note that the white major-ity had shrunk nearly 3 percent (see Figure 2.1).

Most of the people who live in this country are immigrants or are descendants of immigrants. The early waves of immigrants were pre-

Fig. 2.1   Comparison of 1980 and 1990 Censuses
of the United States

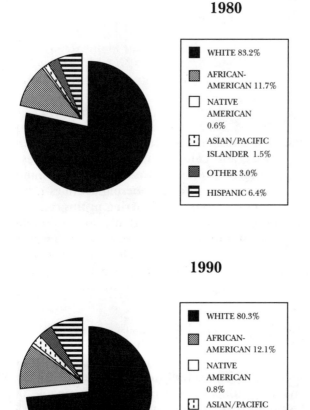

1980

WHITE 83.2%

AFRICAN-
AMERICAN 11.7%

NATIVE
AMERICAN
0.6%

ASIAN/PACIFIC
ISLANDER 1.5%

OTHER 3.0%

HISPANIC 6.4%

1990

WHITE 80.3%

AFRICAN-
AMERICAN 12.1%

NATIVE
AMERICAN
0.8%

ASIAN/PACIFIC
ISLANDER 2.9%

OTHER 3.9%

HISPANIC 9%

Reprinted with permission from Barringer, F. "Census Shows Profound Change in Racial Makeup of Nation." *The New York Times,* March 11, 1991, p. 1.

dominantly European, with subsequent waves coming from Asia during the 1970s and 1980s and presently from Latin America, especially Mexico and Central America (Lefcowitz 1990). The relevance of these population changes to the study of sociocultural aspects of prevention is readily understood, as much of the American norm vis-à-vis prevention is predicated on European philosophies. Every immigrant group has brought its own culture, beliefs, and attitudes. This construct holds for beliefs and practices related to illness prevention as well. A person learns from one's heritage how to maintain health and prevent illness.

Social Barriers to Preventive Health Care

There are innumerable social barriers that prevent people from fully using preventive health services. The overriding barrier is poverty because it restricts access to preventive services. Poverty is more than the mere absence of money. One way of analyzing the phenomenon is to describe the effects of the cycle of poverty. A family in poverty lives in a situation that creates poor intellectual and physical development, poor economic production, and a high birth rate. This situation leads to low productivity, which creates insufficient salaries and a subsistence economy. Poor families must reside in densely populated areas where there is often a lack of shelter and potable water and where they suffer from chronically poor nutrition. These phenomena lead to a high morbidity rate, which precipitates high health care costs that prevent people from seeking preventive services. The resulting increase in sickness and low productivity completes the unending cycle (Spector 1979). Other barriers that are offshoots of this cycle are the lack of access to preventive services, and transportation and language issues.

Cultural Barriers to Preventive Health Care

There are many ways to analyze the role that culture plays in preventive health care practices. This chapter discusses it in the context of heritage consistency and traditional preventive practices. "Heritage consistency," a theory originally developed to provide a means of assessing and counseling Native American alcoholics within a cultural context (Estes and Zitzow 1980), describes "the degree to which one's lifestyle reflects his/her tribal culture." The theory has been expanded in an attempt to study the degree to which a person's life style reflects his/her traditional culture, be it European, Asian, African, or Hispanic. The value characteristics—language of preference, food preferences, name, schools attended, neighborhood ties, and social activities—indicate heritage consistency on a continuum. A person can possess value characteristics of both a heritage-consistent (traditional) and a heritage-inconsistent (acculturated) nature. The concept includes a determination of one's cultural, ethnic, and religious background (Spector 1991). This theory encompasses the following three broad concepts:

1. Culture—the sum total of socially inherited characteristics of a human group that comprises everything that one generation can tell, convey, or hand down to the next (Spector 1991, pp. 50–51).
2. Ethnicity—the condition of belonging to a particular ethnic group. The characteristics of an ethnic group include common language and dialect; race; religious faith or faiths; ties that transcend kinship; neighborhood and community boundaries; and shared traditions, values, and symbols. There are at least 106 different ethnic groups in America and more than 170 Native American tribes or nations (Spector 1991, pp. 51–53).
3. Religion—the belief in superhuman power or powers that must be obeyed and worshipped as the creator(s) and ruler(s) of the universe. It is a system of beliefs, practices, and ethical values. Religion provides a frame of reference and a perspective with which to organize information. Religious teachings vis-à-vis prevention, health, and illness help to present a meaningful philosophy within a system of beliefs, practices, and social controls that have specific values, norms, and ethics and vary among religious groups (Spector 1991, pp. 53–54).

Traditional Beliefs

Numerous beliefs about prevention are manifested by members of the various ethnic communities in the United States. The range of health definitions, beliefs, and practices is infinite, for there are individual differences both within a given group of people and between groups. However, there are also some discernible commonalities in the connotation of the term "health" (see Table 2.1).

Among people who have maintained traditional belief systems, culturally based or "folk" beliefs tend to determine the definitions of health and illness. Folk medicine is related to other types of medicine practiced in our society. It has coexisted, with increasing tensions, with "modern" medicine and was derived from earlier theories of academic medicine. There is ample evidence that folk practices of ancient times have only in part been abandoned in favor of modern belief systems; many continue to be observed today. There are two varieties of folk

Table 2.1 Cross-Cultural Comparison of Selected Connotations of Health, Selected Preventive Practices, and Cultural Phenomena

Nation/Culture of Origin	Health Connotations	Preventive Practices	Communication	Space	Time Orientation
AFRICAN West Coast (as slaves) Many African countries Dominican Republic Jamaica	Harmony of body, mind, and spirit with nature	Religious observances; cleanliness; avoidance of sick people	National languages, dialect, pidgin, Creole, Spanish, French	Close personal space	Present
ASIAN China Hawaii Philippines Korea Japan Southeast Asia Laos Cambodia Vietnam	Balance of Yin and Yang; spiritual and physical harmony with nature	Proper diet, balance of Yin and Yang; jade amulets	National language preference dialects, written characters; use of silence; nonverbal and contextual cuing	Non-contact	Present
EUROPEAN Germany England Italy Ireland Other European countries	Physical and emotional well-being; feeling good	Cleanliness; faith in God	National languages; many learned English immediately	Non-contact; aloof; distant; in southern countries, closer contact and touch	
NATIVE AMERICAN 170 Native American tribes Aleuts Eskimos	Living in harmony with nature	Avoidance of evil spirits; respect for own body and earth	Tribal languages; use of silence and body language	Space is very important and has no boundaries	Present
HISPANIC Spain Cuba Mexico Central and South America	Reward for good behavior; balance "hot and cold"; result of "good luck"	Amulets; prayer; proper balance in diet; avoidance of eclipses	Spanish or Portuguese primary languages	Tactile relationships, touch, handshakes; embracing; physical presence is valued	

medicine: natural folk medicine, or the use of the natural environment—herbs, plants, minerals, and animal substances—to prevent illnesses; and magico-religious folk medicine, or the use of charms, holy
words, and holy actions to prevent illnesses (Spector 1991).

Folk methods of prevention rest in the ability to understand the
cause of a given illness, and beliefs regarding the cause of illness vastly
differ from the modern model of epidemiology. To more fully appreciate the richness of the methods used to prevent illness, it is important
to have an awareness of "traditional epidemiology":

- Traditional agents include hexs, spells, and the "evil eye." Belief in
  the evil eye is one of the oldest beliefs and asserts that there is a
  power that emanates from the eye or mouth that strikes a victim
  with an injury, illness, or other misfortune (Spector 1991). Illness
  may also be caused by people, such as witches, who have the ability
  to make others ill.
- Traditional host factors include phenomena such as "soul loss";
  spirit possession; the ability to provoke the envy, hate, and jealousy
  of a friend, acquaintance, or neighbor, and the religious and social behavior of the subject person. Health is often viewed as the
  reward for "good behavior."
- Traditional environmental factors include air quality ("*mal aire*"),
  and such natural events as a solar eclipse.

Traditional Practices

Traditional practices of prevention developed from folk beliefs about
the causes of illness. People avoided those who were known to cause or
transmit hexs and spells, and many elaborate methods were developed
to counter the envy, hate, and jealousy of others. Countless methods
evolved over generations and still exist today to protect people from
the evil eye. Every effort is made by the host to avoid situations in
which behavior, be it social or religious, is compromised. In many traditions, people take extra precautions to protect themselves from the
mal aire, and pregnant women are not allowed to go outside during an
eclipse.

The following are examples of traditional practices used in the prevention of illness, and others are listed in Table 2.1.

Protective Objects

Various protective objects may be worn, carried, or displayed in the
home. Amulets are objects thought to have magical powers or charms,

and worn on a string or chain around the neck, wrist, or waist to protect the wearer from the evil eye or evil spirits. These spirits could be transmitted from one person to another, or they may have supernatural origins. Amulets are used in societies all over the world and are associated with protection from trouble. In addition to amulets, talismans are consecrated religious objects that wearers believe possess extraordinary powers. The evil eye may also be prevented by touching a baby when it is admired (a Puerto Rican belief), or by drawing a circle around a baby's bed and spitting on the child three times (an Eastern Europe belief).

Substances

This practice employs the use of diet and involves many different observances. It is believed that the body is kept in balance or harmony by the type of food one eats and there are numerous food taboos and combinations that are prescribed in traditional belief systems. People from many ethnic backgrounds eat raw garlic or onion in an effort to prevent illness. Garlic or onions may also be worn on the body or displayed in the home.

Religious Practices

Religion strongly affects the way people choose to prevent illness, and it plays a strong role in rituals associated with prevention. Religion dictates social, moral, and dietary practices that are designed to keep a person in balance and healthy, and plays a vital role in a person's perception of the prevention of illness. Many people believe that illness is prevented by strict adherence to religious codes, morals, and practices and they view illness as a punishment for breaking a religious code.

Other Cultural Considerations

Giger and Davidhizar (1991) identified several factors which vary between cultural groups and are related to the delivery of preventive care (see Table 2.1).

Communication

Communication differences are manifested in the following ways:

- Use of English as the common language.
- Various connotations and denotations for a given word.
- Verbal versus nonverbal communication.
- Use of body language.

Space

The distances that people prefer to keep between one another is a legendary difference among cultural groups. Touch, a source of communication within a spatial relationship, also differs cross-culturally. In some Hispanic cultures, one is expected to shake hands and it is permissible to embrace a person with whom you have a limited acquaintance. In Northern European cultures, this practice is taboo and a touch can do more harm than good. Eye contact is common among people with European backgrounds; people may think the worst when a person does not look them in the eye. Among African-Americans, however, eye contact quite often is taboo.

Time Orientation

Time has countless sets of meanings, two of which are important in the health context. People focus on either specific points in time—clock time, or future orientation—and social time, or present orientation. People who are oriented to the future tend to adhere strictly to clock time. Those who are present-oriented tend not to adhere to rigid time boundaries.

Implications for Community Health Nursing

Nurses practicing in the field of community health must continuously enhance their sensitivity to the cultural needs of clients and their families. An awareness of culturally based health traditions with respect to prevention must be a part of the nurse's early socialization. There must be an ongoing awareness of changing demographic and immigration trends, as well as continuous monitoring of social and political responses to issues such as poverty and homelessness. Whenever possible, an ability to communicate in another language must be fostered, either by speaking it or using interpreters. Community health nurses must be aware of a person's perception of space and time orientation. These are several of the sustaining activities that will enhance the cross-cultural practice of community health nursing.

References

Barringer, F. 1991, March 11. Census shows profound change in racial makeup of the nation. *The New York Times*, p. 1.

Estes, G., and Zitzow, D. 1980. Heritage consistency as a consideration in counseling Native Americans. Paper presented at the National Indian Education Association Convention, Dallas.

Giger, J. N., and Davidhizar, R. E. 1991. *Transcultural nursing assessment and inter-*

vention. St. Louis: Mosby Year Book.

Lefcowitz, E. 1990. *The United States immigration history timeline.* New York: Terra Firma Press.

Sege, I., and Mashek, J. 1991. Census total will stand despite undercounting. *The Boston Globe,* p. 1.

Spector, M. 1979. Poverty: The barrier to health care. In *Cultural diversity in health and illness,* R. Spector, ed., pp. 141–162. New York: Appleton, Century, and Crofts.

Spector, R. 1991. *Cultural diversity in health and illness,* 3rd ed. Norwalk, CT: Appleton & Lang.

3

Establishing Community Coalitions for Prevention: Healthy Cities Indiana

Beverly C. Flynn, Ph.D., R.N., F.A.A.N.
Professor, Department of Community Health Nursing,
Indiana University School of Nursing, Indianapolis, Indiana;
Director, Institute of Action Research for Community Health;
Head, World Health Organization Collaborating Center in Healthy Cities; and
Director, CITYNET Healthy Cities

and

Joanne W. Rains, D.N.Sc., R.N.
Assistant Professor, Department of Community Health Nursing,
Indiana University School of Nursing, Indianapolis, Indiana;
Fellow, Institute of Action Research for Community Health;
Fellow, World Health Organization Collaborating Center in Healthy Cities

"History teaches us that organized community effort to prevent disease and promote health is both valuable and effective."
(Institute of Medicine 1988, p. 17)

Prevention is rarely a solo endeavor. Even when it originates as an individual choice and action, prevention can be traced to an enabling policy or a supportive structure. This is especially true at the community level.

One form of community action is the formation of coalitions for health promotion or prevention of disease. These coalitions are gatherings of diverse entities focusing their resources and efforts on some common goal. Examples of community coalitions are abundant, and include one innovation, the Healthy Cities Indiana project.

This chapter uses the Healthy Cities model to illustrate the potential for community coalitions to prevent disease and promote health. Included are discussions on the theoretical understanding of coalitions, the Healthy Cities model, and examples of unique community coalitions (or theory in practice). The chapter concludes by describing the Healthy Cities Indiana coalition as an example of primary prevention at the community level.

Theoretical Understanding of Coalitions

Community coalitions are diverse groups and individuals who join together to accomplish goals they are unable or unlikely to achieve individually. Coalitions involve temporary alliances; they function only to work toward an unmet goal that is relevant to the membership. "Temporary" also implies that coalitions can expand their membership or move on to new agendas or redefine their purpose as needs and interest change. Coalitions are instruments of change.

Most of the literature on coalitions is theoretical, with little agreement on the most useful theory. Examples of the various theories include game theory, social psychological models, and political or power models (Murninghan 1978). In the absence of a unifying theory, we can list and describe some concepts common to each:

- *Payoffs:* the value or benefit for those involved. Individual coalition members try to maximize their payoffs, while pursuing the common goal.
- *Resources:* the cost of what one brings to the coalition. Resources can determine members' relative degree of control.
- *Shared Ideology:* similar views or notions that contribute to similar goals and desired outcomes.

The context for these three concepts is usually instability, change, or scarcity. These conditions propel groups to work together rather than compete for finite resources and a place on the political agenda.

In contrast to the theoretical writings, Dluhy (1990) presents practical help in building and maintaining coalitions. The complex social problems encountered at the community level present challenges best met by a comprehensive approach that cuts across agency, service, or turf boundaries. Coalitions facilitate that comprehensive approach, promote innovation, and maximize scarce community resources. The whole of a productive coalition exceeds the sum of its parts.

Dluhy (1990) discusses two kinds of functions served by coalitions: task-oriented and interpersonal. The task-oriented function relates to a coalition as an instrument of change. The desired outcomes can be non-political goals, such as community education on a particular issue, or social networking for support and idea exchange. The desired outcomes also can be political goals, such as obtaining financial resources or other public policy action within government. Examples of political goals are securing a portion of tax money for a child care clinic, or passing an ordinance banning smoking in public places. Political goals are central to community coalitions for prevention.

Community credibility and timing are two features crucial to task-oriented functions. The coalition must be perceived as an expert and appropriate voice, and it must speak at the appropriate time. Timing within the policy arena involves recognizing and maximizing those brief moments when the windows of opportunity are open.

Interpersonal functions deal with building and maintaining coalition membership. Diverse membership requires a leader who is flexible, capable of managing conflict and change, and able to articulate the vision across disciplines or agencies. To be successful, coalitions also need an internal consensus-building process. Communication is vital to receiving membership input, developing a shared direction, and keeping people focused on the agenda.

Coalitions, therefore, are instruments of change. They focus the diverse resources of individuals or community groups to accomplish political and non-political goals.

Healthy Cities Model

The Healthy Cities Movement

Healthy Cities began in 1986 as a project of the European Region of the World Health Organization(WHO). It was an outgrowth of an international conference on health promotion in Ottawa, Ontario, Canada. Though original plans included five to eight project cities, in just over five years, there is a network of over 30 European project cities, 17 national, and three international networks encompassing hundreds of cities throughout the world (Tsouros 1990).

The Healthy Cities project places health high on the city's political agenda. Cities are simultaneously involved in developing and implementing specific plans to improve health in the city and taking the necessary steps to obtain the resources to make these plans possible. Key city challenges include reducing inequalities in health status in the population; developing healthy public policies at the local level; creating physical and social environments that support health; strengthening community action for health; helping people develop new skills for health; and reorienting health services to be supportive of the principles of health promotion and the concepts of health for all by the year 2000. The mayors and top political representatives of the project cities have issued a strong declaration of political support, and a number of cities have allocated significant resources to the project. The project has established new partnerships for health and has paved the way for a new European public health movement (Tsouros 1990).

Clearly, the Healthy Cities project has become a worldwide social movement aimed at social change in health promotion and primary prevention of disease. As a social movement, Healthy Cities also exemplifies major concepts of coalition behavior. Community health is a shared ideology of diverse groups, all of which can maximize their payoffs while pursuing common goals. Application of the Health Cities model in the United States, and particularly in Indiana, expands our understanding of coalition behavior.

The Indiana Model: A Shared Ideology

As successful as Healthy Cities has been in Europe, political and philosophical differences between the United States and Europe require adaptations of the plan to this country. In addition, public health in the United States has been characterized as being in disarray, lacking the power needed to pursue essential programs (Institute of Medicine 1988). Local cities are faced with expanded responsibilities for health without the added resources necessary. City leaders need new approaches that will help them with these conditions of change and scarce resources.

Healthy Cities Indiana establishes community coalitions for primary prevention through shared ideology, emphasizing a community development approach to decision making in health. This approach assumes that public policies are improved through citizen participation in the policy making process. The Indiana model of Healthy Cities seeks to assist local communities in developing leadership for broad-based solutions to today's complex health concerns.

Six cities are participating in Healthy Cities Indiana: Fort Wayne, Gary, Indianapolis, Jeffersonville, New Castle, and Seymour. The cities are scattered throughout the state and represent both rural and urban areas.

The shared ideology necessary for community coalitions includes the following objectives:

- Put health first on the public agenda.
- Share responsibility for health community-wide.
- Involve local people.
- Focus on hard-to-reach populations.
- Promote healthy public policies.

The Indiana model of Healthy Cities involves the following factors to achieve these objectives:

- City commitment demonstrated by both the local health officer and mayor.
- Establishment of a Healthy City committee that is broadly representative of the community.
- A commitment that health is defined broadly and involves participation by all sectors of the community.
- Development of leadership for health within the city.
- Community assessments and a public debate about the health of the community.

- Identification of health problems and strengths in the community.
- Development of solutions to problems community-wide.
- Mutual support, collaboration, and shared learning among the six cities.
- Provision of data-based information to policy makers, information upon which healthy public policies can be built.
- Monitoring and evaluating of Healthy City projects over time.
- Sharing of information with others interested in developing a healthy city.

Costs and Benefits to the Cities: Resources and Payoffs

Because of a grant from the W.K. Kellogg Foundation, participation in Healthy Cities Indiana required no direct financing by the city or participating organizations. The grant covers consultation with people who have experience in implementing a Healthy City program; workshops, conferences, and network sessions that help community leaders analyze existing information and local surveys; establishing a vision for a Healthy City; delineating Healthy City plans and action strategies; working with the media and policy makers; securing resources for Healthy Cities; and monitoring and evaluating Healthy City progress.

One of the intended outcomes of the Indiana model of Healthy Cities is to develop a process to ensure that the health of citizens becomes a prime factor in public and political decision making. As noted earlier, this process requires a commitment by city leaders to community-wide, broad-based participation in Healthy Cities. City leaders, public health departments, and local citizens participate in assessing the broader health needs of the community, local public policies' impact on health, and the solutions to community health problems. Participating in Healthy Cities requires energy to see such a commitment through, whatever political processes may be required.

What does a city get for its expenditure of money, energy, commitment, and time?

- Community leaders who have developed their skills in the Healthy City process.
- A constituency for public health capable of addressing complex community health problems.
- A network within and across cities that is taking action on solutions that work locally.
- The development of healthy public policies that focus on health promotion and disease prevention.

Unique Community Coalitions

Central to the implementation of Healthy Cities is the formation of a broad-based coalition, the Healthy City committee. Committee members are selected by the mayor and public health officer with input from local citizens as well as agencies and organizations that support the Healthy City concept. The committee consists of community leaders from different sectors of city life, including arts/culture, business/industry, dentistry, education, employment, environment, finance, health and medical care, local government, media, parks/recreation, planning/housing, population groups, public health, religion, social services, transportation, and utilities/energy. Committee members do not represent a particular sector of the community per se, but serve to bring the perspective of that sector to the Healthy City committee and facilitate the communication of ideas and actions between the sector and the committee.

The six Healthy City committees were established in 1989 and they each have taken action to identify and receive the input of local residents, particularly the under-represented. This outreach has included establishing action subcommittees, conducting community vision workshops and forums, and conducting population and community-wide surveys.

What has been accomplished in the Healthy Cities since 1989? Each of the cities has been involved in taking short-term action and devising long-range strategies aimed at community health promotion and disease prevention. The smaller or rural cities have been able to mobilize faster than the larger cities in metropolitan areas. The problems and structure of organizations are usually not as complex in smaller communities, and the local network for action can be more easily tapped.

The Healthy Cities examples presented below exemplify the two functions of coalitions discussed by Dluhy (1990): the task-oriented and the interpersonal. The examples suggest the Healthy City committees have been instruments of change in their communities. Through their action they have gained credibility in the community and are learning the importance of timing their strategies to maximize results. The interpersonal activities of the Healthy City committees have centered on building and maintaining the coalition membership. The chairs and co-chairs of the Healthy City committees are promoting consensus through communication and developing a shared direction at committee meetings.

Rural Areas

The first city to take action was in a rural area. A dentist on the Healthy City committee observed a number of mouth injuries among children who participated in contact sports. Following an analysis of local information and the literature, the committee decided to institute a mouth guard campaign for youths participating in contact sports during the summer months. The mayor, who was an active member of the Healthy City committee, contacted the manager of the local pharmacy and obtained the pharmacy's cosponsorship of the campaign, along with discounts for youths who purchased the mouth guards. A media campaign was launched that gave excellent coverage of the mouth guard campaign and enhanced the Healthy City committee's image in the community.

On one hand, the campaign was a success; it made a positive statement to the community about the Healthy City committee's concern with injury prevention. On the other hand, however, the children did not wear the mouth guards. The committee decided that the children themselves needed to be more involved in this decision, so members scheduled group meetings with the children to hear their reasons for not wearing the mouth guards and to explain the intent of the campaign. The committee also decided to promote a policy change so that all children would be required to wear mouth guards during contact sports. Efforts are underway to promote healthy public policy through the state high-school sports regulatory commission and through the dental association. This effort, which started as a short-term action, has evolved into a long-range prevention strategy.

Another rural city identified some environmental problems. Children reported that the streets were dirty and the adults agreed. The mayor's office reported that it would be difficult to recruit new business unless the issue of solid waste management was addressed. As a short-term action, the Healthy City committee collaborated with other organizations and supported a city street clean-up project. This project increased civic pride among participants and empowered the committee to work on a recycling effort. A recycling day was so successful that the city has worked on establishing recycling bins in several areas of the city. The committee also has realized that decision making in environmental health rests with the district solid-waste management advisory committee. The Healthy City committee has identified and recommended appropriate community members to serve on this committee.

Another rural city decided that its problems and strengths extended beyond the city boundaries into the county. The city recently reorganized its Healthy City committee to include Healthy Communities in the county. With this expanded coalition in place, the committee has been working diligently on establishing a primary health-care clinic for low-income families in the county. Members are mobilizing local physicians, the health department, the hospital, and others to work together in creating a plan that will work locally. Currently, the committee is pursuing funding from a foundation to employ a nurse practitioner to develop the clinic.

Metropolitan Areas

One large city discovered that most of its crimes occur between 5:00
a.m. and 7:00 a.m. In exploring solutions to this problem, the Healthy
City committee decided to develop a project that involves the city's
waste haulers and police. The project is designed to train city refuse
collectors to be neighborhood crime watchers and report suspicious
activity to the police using their truck radios.

Another large city found that it needed more community input into
decision making. The Healthy City committee decided to hold a "Vi-
sions of Healthy City Poster Contest" with school children in grades
four through twelve. The committee obtained cosponsorship from a
local business that paid for the prizes for the winning youths and their
schools. After the contest, the business was so pleased with the winning
posters that they paid for them to be printed as holiday greeting cards.
The committee also conducted vision workshops for thirty-three neighborhood associations: they were invited to bring local citizens, including youths, to discuss their ideas about what their city would be like if
it were a Healthy City.

The results of these projects were summarized by the Healthy Cities
staff and shared with the Healthy City committee for its deliberations,
resulting in the formation of five action subcommittees. At the same
time, two of the neighborhood associations became interested in the
Healthy Cities process and requested that project staff work with them
in developing Healthy Neighborhoods. This city now has Healthy City
coalition activities occurring at two levels—neighborhood and city. Although the activities of each are parallel and independent, communication between these two levels occurs through the city-wide Healthy
City committee and through project staff.

The third large city identified multiple problems in their city including substance abuse, a lack of civic pride, and high unemployment, especially among young people. The Healthy City committee decided to
initiate a summer "Walk Against Drugs" for youths ages six to fourteen
years. The event drew close to 500 participants who walked the one-
mile course, browsed through six health information booths located in
strategic points along the walk, and received a special preview of the
career and hobby exposition. During the walk, the committee sur-
veyed all the youth walkers' knowledge and use of various drugs. The
committee considered the event a success and plans to involve more
citizens, community groups, and children in this year's event.

The Healthy Cities Indiana Network: Expanding the Coalition

As the cities develop their ideas, they learn from the other Healthy
Cities. For example, members of one Healthy City committee have

been invited to present at another Healthy City committee meeting on managing solid waste. The cities have learned from each other by making site visits to other cities; by participating in network sessions, where one of the Healthy Cities hosts the others; and through *CITYNET*, the quarterly Healthy Cities Indiana newsletter.

As a step in placing Healthy Cities on the state's political agenda, the six Healthy Cities helped to develop and support a resolution, "Promoting Healthy Cities in Indiana." The resolution was filed for consideration by one of the Healthy City's senators in the 1990 Indiana General Assembly and passed both the House of Representatives and the Senate to become public policy. The passage of the resolution is significant because it represents the first successful collective step of the Healthy Cities coalition in influencing state policy.

Over the years, the Healthy Cities Indiana project office has received hundreds of requests for Healthy Cities information and placement on the *CITYNET* mailing list. In recognition of the work of Healthy Cities Indiana, the Indiana University School of Nursing Institute of Action Research for Community Health was designated as a WHO Collaborating Center in Healthy Cities. This designation provides new opportunities in Healthy Cities research, training, and practice, expanding the coalition globally.

Healthy Cities Coalitions as Primary Prevention

The Institute of Medicine (1988) defends the contribution that public health has made to the health status of the nation, citing maternal/child programs or control of infectious diseases as only two examples. This study repeatedly emphasizes that the approaches needed for current health challenges are organized and sustained efforts by the public. "Public health . . . involves 'organized community effort.' It is not simply the outcome of isolated individual efforts. Its mission is to ensure that organized approaches are mobilized when they are needed" (p. 39). Through coalitions like the Healthy Cities committee, the public can, in a coordinated manner, pursue health.

The coalition approach is well-suited for complex problems that require community-level solutions, and is required when there is competition for scarce resources. Coalitions, therefore, are appropriate vehicles for the prevention of disease and the promotion of health in today's environment.

Coalitions perform task-oriented and interpersonal functions. From a prevention perspective, the most important function involves task-oriented political goals. Political goals pertinent to prevention include getting health on the political agenda, receiving funding for public health, and influencing the creation of healthy public policy.

Healthy Cities Indiana is as an example of establishing community coalitions for preventive health. The Healthy Cities committee shared the vision of living in a healthy city, and joined resources and efforts to educate and influence policy makers toward this end. Public policy shapes the choices we can make as a community. By working to influence these policies, a community coalition can be engaged in primary prevention in its purest form.

References

Dluhy, M.J. 1990. *Building coalitions in the human services*. Newbury Park, CA: Sage.

Institute of Medicine. 1988. *The future of public health*. Washington, DC: National Academy Press.

Murninghan, J. 1978. Models of coalition behavior: Game theoretic, social pyschological and political perspective. *Psychological Bulletin* 85, 1130–1163.

Tsouros, A.D. 1990. *World Health Organization Healthy Cities Project: A project becomes a movement*. Copenhagen: FADL Publishers.

4

Prevention: Maternal and Infant Health

Judith McFarlane, Dr. P.H., R.N., F.A.A.N.
Director, De Madres a Madres
Director, Abuse during Pregnancy
Professor
College of Nursing
Texas Woman's University
Houston, Texas

and

Carol Patwari, B.S.N., R.N.
Program Coordinator
Community Health Nurse
Harris County Health Department
Houston, Texas

Cindy, a 28-year-old college graduate, is excited about her long-awaited, recently confirmed first pregnancy of nine weeks. Despite her husband's unemployment and violent behavior, Cindy is sure everything will be fine once the baby arrives. Knowing the importance of early prenatal care, Cindy wants to initiate health care immediately. However, without health insurance, her private health-care provider is no longer an option. Fortified with education, English proficiency, and her determination to have a healthy pregnancy, Cindy makes her first phone call to gain access to early prenatal care.

Twenty-one-year-old Maria just arrived via car trunk from her war-ravaged country to begin a better life with her husband, José. Pregnant with her third child, Maria will try to conceal her pregnancy and seek work alongside José, an unskilled laborer, so they can send money back home to care for their other two children, who are too young to make the arduous trip. Neither Maria nor José speaks English. Although she is very concerned about her baby, Maria is in no hurry to make her presence known by attempting to access prenatal care. Besides, as she tells José, "Both of our children were born fat and healthy and I never saw a doctor."

Tina, age 16 years, six months pregnant and unmarried, does not know when or with whom the pregnancy began. Addicted to cocaine and existing from high to high, Tina wonders how she will get money for more drugs. When asked about the pregnancy, Tina averts her eyes and walks away.

Mothers and Infants at Risk

Worldwide, half a million women die each year as a result of pregnancy or childbirth-related causes (WHO 1990). In industrialized countries, the figures vary from one woman per 4,000 to one woman per 10,000. Every one of these deaths is preventable. In the United States, African-American mothers die at three times the rate of white women and African-American infants are far more likely to die during the first twelve months of life than non-African-American infants (DHHS 1990). Birth weight is the leading determinant of infant health; children with low birth weight are at increased risk of mortality, morbidity, and lifelong neurodevelopmental handicaps (Institute of Medicine 1988).

Although early prenatal care is essential for maternal and infant health, one-third of all pregnant women do not receive adequate care. For mothers who begin prenatal care during the first trimester, infant mortality rates are 9.7 per 1,000. For mothers without prenatal care, infant mortality is 48.7 per 1,000. Prenatal care reduces the risk of mortality fivefold and ensures the health of mother and child (Torres and Kenney 1989). Prenatal care is also cost-effective. Each dollar spent on prenatal care for high-risk women saves $3.38 in medical care for a low birth-weight infant. Smoking, substance abuse, poor nutrition, infection, anemia, and toxemia are all associated with low birth weight, and each is amenable to intervention through early prenatal care.

The United States has set forth objectives for healthy mothers and infants for the year 2000 which set the goal that 90 percent of all pregnant women would begin prenatal care within the first three months of pregnancy. Based on the latest available figures, the nation will not meet the goal until the year 2094, nearly 100 years after the target date (Children's Defense Fund 1989). Lack of insurance, fear, ambivalence, past experiences with the health care system, customs, beliefs, and life style practices all contribute to a reluctance to get early care.

In some Spanish-speaking cultures, pregnancy is viewed as a normal process, modesty is highly valued, and family support and female care providers are the norm. It is unlikely that a woman from such a culture would be eager to enter a clinic to be examined by a male physician with whom she cannot communicate. Without private insurance, she would need to complete reams of paperwork to establish financial eligibility. She would frequently shuttle between several offices, and almost always have to wait. It is easy to understand why, having gone through such a process once, during subsequent pregnancies this woman would choose to begin care late or not at all.

Health objectives for the year 2000 contain 14 priority health care objectives relating to maternal and infant health (DHHS 1990). The objectives focus on decreasing infant and maternal mortality, fetal deaths, fetal alcohol syndrome, low birth weight, complications of pregnancy, and caesarean-section delivery rates. The objectives also focus on health promotion; recommended weight gain; breast-feeding levels; abstinence from tobacco, alcohol, and drugs; and early access to prenatal care, along with screening and counseling for fetal abnormalities. How will the nation make these objectives a reality?

Efforts to Date

Medicaid was enacted in 1965 to provide health care to low-income individuals. It is the largest single source of health care financing for the poor in the United States. In recent years, in an effort to reduce infant mortality, Congress has expanded Medicaid guidelines to provide a broader range of coverage for pregnant women and their infants. Originally, eligibility was limited to women receiving cash assistance through Aid to Families with Dependent Children (AFDC) and Social Security programs. As a result, poor, married women and single women pregnant with their first child were excluded.

In 1984, changes were made to include these two groups if they fell within poverty guidelines. In 1987, linkage with cash-assisted programs was dropped. Congress mandated that by July 1990 states must cover women and infants up to 100 percent of the poverty level. An estimated 361,000 pregnant women were now eligible for Medicaid (Torres and Kenney 1989). Will these women enroll? Will this policy result in increases in early prenatal care and healthier mothers and infants?

Probably not. There is a paucity of outreach and effective communication to inform women of their eligibility for Medicaid. Once informed, the eligibility process is cumbersome and discourages enrollment. For those who persist, the process often takes several trips to the screening office, securing various personal documents (such as birth certificate and residency status), written pregnancy confirmation, and a waiting period of a month or more.

The eligibility process almost certainly precludes starting prenatal care in the first trimester. Measures such as presumptive eligibility help speed the process, but not all states have adopted this system. In addition, 44 percent of physicians who provide obstetrical services will not accept Medicaid clients, leaving the pregnant woman with no recourse but to turn to the public health clinics, which are already understaffed and unable in most cases to direct the woman to a clinic during the first trimester. Although expansion of Medicaid is essential to improve maternal and infant health, without concurrent community outreach, information dissemination, and rapid eligibility processing, the journey to accessing early prenatal care will remain difficult and lengthy.

Once the woman secures a prenatal appointment, other support programs become more accessible, the largest being the Special Supplemental Food Program for Women, Infants, and Children (WIC). WIC is a supplemental nutrition program, federally sponsored, that serves low-income pregnant and postpartum women, and children who are nutritionally at risk. The program provides coordination of health care resources, nutrition education, and food supplements. Enrollment is meant to improve pregnancy outcomes as well as promote children's physical growth and cognitive development.

In the largest national longitudinal study to evaluate the impact of WIC, no evidence was found that WIC enrollment affects the frequency of prenatal care, rate of breast-feeding, level of alcohol and tobacco use, or any statistically significant decrease in fetal mortality (Rush et al. 1988). Positive associations were found for reversal of low weight gain in early pregnancy, increased intake of key nutrients, decreased premature rupture of membranes, thirty- to sixty-gram increase in birth weight, and larger infant head circumference. As with other programs, WIC alone cannot solve all the problems related to maternal and infant health. Creative and innovative programs are needed that focus on removing barriers for the individual woman and simultaneously increasing the accessibility of prenatal care. We know early prenatal care works—we do not know how to make it more accessible.

Partnerships for Prevention

De Madres a Madres: A Community Partnership for Health

Compared to non-Hispanic white and African-American women, Hispanic women are the least likely to receive early prenatal care. In Houston, the fourth largest city in the nation, 70 percent of pregnant women initiate prenatal care during the first trimester; for Hispanic women the figure falls to 61 percent. Hispanics are the fastest-growing aggregate in America. Improving access to prenatal care for Hispanic women will have a major impact on meeting the Surgeon General's goals for the nation.

Barriers to accessing prenatal care have been discussed. For the Hispanic woman, additional barriers of language and immigration status present major obstacles to beginning care. Based on concepts of community partnerships, volunteerism, and empowerment of women, an inner-city Hispanic community in Houston was targeted for an intervention project called De Madres a Madres: A Community Partnership for Health ("de madres a madres" means "from mothers to mothers" in Spanish). The program consists of volunteer mothers offering culturally relevant social support and information on community resources to high-risk women in their community. The goal of providing referral information and support empowers the women, thereby improving access to early prenatal care. The target community consists of two census tracts that contain a population of 13,555; of these, 34 percent are women of childbearing age. The median family income is $12,782, and 19 percent of the households receive public assistance.

De Madres a Madres was begun with modest seed-grant funds from the local March of Dimes. One community health nurse completed a community assessment to identify community leaders, who were visited individually and apprised of the program's goals and objectives. Each community leader was asked to provide names of potential volunteer mothers. (Since most community leaders were men, sharing the names of women yielded an endorsement for the program from the male hierarchy.) At the same time, formal presentations about the program were made at scheduled community functions, including school, civic, and church meetings, as well as informal presentations at bazaars, fiestas, and health fairs. At each presentation, the importance of early prenatal care was stressed, and the idea of volunteer mothers reaching out to at-risk mothers to offer concern and community resource information was presented.

Mothers responded, and at the end of nine months, 14 volunteers had completed the eight-hour training session with the community health nurse. The mothers varied in age from 19 years to 68 years, and held a variety of positions within the community. For example, several of the volunteer mothers worked at the church pantry, two were elementary school secretaries, one was a laundromat attendant, two were clerks at the local grocery, one was a waitress, another was a bank receptionist, one was the president of the high school PTA, and several were esteemed grandmothers and great-grandmothers. Because of their positions, the volunteer mothers came into contact daily with mothers who were at-risk of not starting early prenatal care.

In a typical situation, a pregnant mother arrives at her child's elementary school and is greeted by a volunteer mother and asked about her pregnancy. The volunteer mother offers community resource information and a follow-up phone call or home visit. Frequently, at the home visit the volunteer mother learns of additional family concerns such as ill children, lack of insurance, or a pending eviction. Beginning with the identified needs of the mother, the volunteer mother offers appropriate community referral information and an empathic attitude, and makes arrangements for future visits. The community health nurse talks to the volunteer mothers weekly and frequently accompanies them on home visits.

Many high-risk women are undocumented aliens and unaware of how to obtain prenatal care without reprisal. Many of these women frequent the food pantry in the community where volunteer mothers offer social support and community resource information to 75 to 100 women each week. An additional outreach strategy is to set up information booths at the local grocery store, shopping center, and bank. Local merchants provide a fruit basket, canned ham, or other item for a drawing. The volunteer mothers staff the booth, offering community resource information to interested persons, along with home visitation or a phone call for further information. Everyone who registers for the door prize is asked if she would like more information about the program. Usually 60 to 80 women register; many request a phone call or home visit. All information is in Spanish and all the volunteers are bilingual.

The community formed a partnership with the volunteer mothers, and soon referrals came from all areas of the community. For example, an officer at the community police station noticed a pregnant woman who was accompanying a man requesting information. When the police officer inquired about the pregnancy and health care, the woman shared that she and her family were new to the area and not aware of where to go for health care. The officer informed the pregnant woman about the De Madres a Madres program, offered her a brochure in Spanish, and asked if she would like him to call a volunteer mother. She requested a call, which started her prenatal care.

Although early prenatal care is a primary goal of the program, pregnancy status is never solicited unless it is obvious. The basic premise of De Madres a Madres is primary prevention. Information is power, and if women are provided with culturally relevant information they will use the information when the pregnancy is confirmed. Volunteer mothers are taught that information is empowerment and that contact is success. Women empowered with information will choose when and how to use the information. It is also assumed that women will share the information with relatives, friends, and neighbors, creating a ripple effect throughout the community. Now, women in the community go directly to a De Madres a Madres volunteer mother, saying that they found out about the program from a co-worker, neighbor, friend, or family member, or that they picked up a brochure at the bakery, laundromat, or drugstore.

The safety net for Hispanic women in Houston is growing, a community partnership is solidifying. Community ownership follows community awareness, involvement, and commitment. At the end of the second year of the program, the volunteer mothers had offered information to more than 3,000 women in the community. The W.K. Kellogg Foundation has funded establishment of a center in the community from which the volunteer mothers will offer resource information and social support to a wider community of women. When a volunteer mother who has two children and who works full-time was asked why she donated her time, her reply was quick and sure: "Why would I not help these women? This community is my home. I care about these women."

Violence against Women: A Primary Prevention Model in a Health Care Agency

Violence against women is pervasive. National estimates are that one in two women will be physically assaulted at least once during her lifetime by a man with whom she lives. Many times the battering begins during pregnancy. Physical abuse during pregnancy has recently been recognized as a significant risk to the health of both the mother and infant. Trauma is a complication in 6 percent to 7 percent of all pregnancies, with only 50 percent of the injuries sustained from automobile accidents. When interviewed, 4 percent to 8 percent of pregnant women reported battering during pregnancy, and battered women were more likely to deliver a low birth-weight infant.

In the first national study (*Journal of the American Medical Association* 1992) of 1,200 African-American, white, and Hispanic pregnant women, preliminary data document the occurrence of physical abuse during the past 12 months to be 23 percent—one in four women— and battering during the current pregnancy at 16 percent, one in every six women. A possible reason for the higher reported rate of 16 percent is that the women are interviewed by their primary care nurse, with whom they have probably developed a trusting relationship. In addition, the pregnant women were interviewed three times during pregnancy, and women who denied abuse initially reported abuse later in the pregnancy.

When access to prenatal care was analyzed, 29 percent of the abused women began prenatal care in the third trimester compared to 15 percent of the non-abused women. Physical abuse may be part of a constellation of behaviors detrimental to maternal and infant health, including avoidance of health care forcefully imposed on the woman by the abuser. Assessment of abuse, combined with education, advocacy, and community referral information, is a powerful intervention to prevent violence. In the cited study, 50 percent of the women reporting (abuse during pregnancy) at the first prenatal visit reported no further abuse at the second and third trimester visits.

Many pregnant women have only one prenatal visit. For abused women who begin prenatal care late, there may be only one assessment opportunity and only one chance to relay information on abuse and options to protect the mother and child. The head is a primary target for abuse, and since injuries around the head are readily visible to clinicians as well as the general public, the evidence of the abuse may contribute to missed prenatal visits.

To prevent abuse during pregnancy, special abuse assessment guides, protocols of care, and referral sources exist (McFarlane 1991). Reduction of violent and abusive behavior is a targeted objective for Year 2000 health objectives (DHHS 1990). The Surgeon General has titled battering during pregnancy a "Crime against the Future" and has recommended, along with the American College of Obstetricians and Gynecologists and ANA, that all women be routinely screened for physical abuse and offered a protocol of care. Since pregnancy is the only time that healthy women come into frequent, scheduled contact with nurses, assessment and intervention for abuse during pregnancy provide an opportunity to interrupt and prevent the cycle of violence and protect the health and safety of both mother and infant.

To prevent violence toward women, in one community a partnership was formed between the public health department and the surrounding area. Once the decision was made to institute assessment for abuse as part of the standard prenatal intake data, community resources that assist battered women were contacted and asked to make presentations to the clinic staff, providing introductions to key personnel, hours of operation, services provided, and costs. The information was put into a brochure that was given to clinic staff and eventually to all clients. All information was updated every six months.

The knowledge base for staff education on abuse was crisis intervention. It was stressed that abuse was another crisis with which to combine crisis intervention theory. By definition, crisis is short-term, usually about six weeks. The focus of crisis intervention is present-oriented and directed toward restoration to a pre-crisis level of functioning. The staff dealt daily with minor crises, (e.g., elevated blood glucose, increased blood pressure) and major crises (e.g., no audible fetal heart tones, an ultrasound suggesting congenital anomalies). The staff had adequate knowledge about each of these crises, and coupled their knowledge about the condition with crisis intervention theory to intervene on clients' behalfs. The staff were receptive to knowledge about physical abuse because they had a framework of crisis intervention within which to add the facts and frame an intervention plan.

Assessing for abuse, crisis intervention, and follow-up is emotionally draining work. Staff support was built into the program with the "buddy system," whereby two nurses were assigned to each other as partners. After one of the partners has screened a battered woman or seen a battered woman on a follow-up return visit, the buddy is responsible for taking that staff member aside and stopping for a five-minute debriefing session (preferably over a cup of coffee).

The agency administration can support staff by having a clear understanding of the goal of abuse assessment and crisis intervention. Most people think that the goal is to have the abused woman leave the abusive partner or to have the abuse stop. In reality, most abused women leave and return to the abusive relationship many times. Most battered women want the abuse to end, not the relationship. Many abused women perceive few options and lack the finances to establish another household for themselves and their children. The goal of abuse assessment must be contact with the abused woman. Contact is success; it begins a sharing of information, advocacy, and referral sources and establishes a partnership between the woman and nurse. When a woman answers questions about abuse, she has entrusted the nurse with very private information. A therapeutic relationship has begun; the battered woman will choose when, where, and how to use the information.

Contact plus information equals empowerment. Both the De Madres a Madres program and the abuse assessment initiative focused on prevention partnerships to empower women to act to promote their health and that of their unborn child.

Summary

Community health nurses are the vanguard of prevention, whether in grass roots, community-based or agency-initiated efforts to promote maternal and child health. Health promotion begins with primary prevention. Community health nurses are in a unique position to influence not only the health of today's mothers but that of tomorrow's mothers, who are now infants.

If healthy mothers and infants are to be a reality for the 21st century, then universal access to early prenatal care is imperative. A service delivery system that is culturally responsive and sensitive to individual needs is a must, along with nurses who advocate for women and empower them with resources.

Our present system does not work. Women are not receiving early prenatal care, children are not born with a healthy start. Prevention partnerships between community health nurses and their constituents can make the health objectives for the year 2000 a reality and the journeys of pregnant women successful.

The authors wish to dedicate this chapter to community and public health nurses everywhere who form partnerships for prevention with pregnant women, their unborn children, and the communities within which they reside. Yours is a noble profession.

References

Children's Defense Fund. 1989. *The health of America's children: Maternal and child health data book.* New York: Author.

Institute of Medicine. 1988. *Prenatal care: Reaching mothers, reaching infants.* Washington, DC: National Academy Press.

McFarlane, J. 1991. Battering in pregnancy. In *Violence Against Women: Nursing research, education and practice issues,* Carolyn M. Sampselle ed. New York: Hemisphere Press.

McFarlane, J., Parker, P., Soeken, K., and Bullock, L. 1992. Assessing for abuse during pregnancy: Frequency and extent of injuries and associated entry into prenatal care. *Journal of American Medical Association* 267(23), 3176–3179.

Rush, D., Horvits, D., Seaver, B., Alvir, J., Garbowski, G., Leighton, J., Sloan, N., Johnson, S., Kulka, R., and Shanklin, S. 1988. The national WIC evaluation: Evaluation of the special Supplemental Food Program for Women, Infants, and Children. *American Journal of Clinical Nutrition* 48, 389–393.

Torres A., and Kenney A. 1989. Expanding medicaid coverage for pregnant women: Estimates of the impact and cost. *Family Planning Perspectives* 21(1), 19–24.

U.S. Department of Health and Human Services. 1990. *Healthy people 2000: National health promotion and disease prevention objectives.* Washington, DC: U.S. Government Printing Office.

World Health Organization. 1990. *Facts about WHO.* Geneva: Author.

5

Prevention: Child Health

Judith B. Igoe, M.S., R.N., F.A.A.N.
Associate Professor,
Director, School Health Programs
University of Colorado Health Sciences Center
Denver, Colorado

Preschoolers and school-age youth are the healthiest segment of the American population. They have survived the perils of infancy but have not yet faced the dangers inherent in adolescence nor the degenerative diseases of old age. Most of their illnesses and injuries are preventable if complete immunization, acceptable living conditions, and adequate parenting are provided. Developmentally, these children are eager and ready to learn, making this age group a population ripe for health education and health promotion activities. This chapter reviews the factors that threaten the health of American children and focuses on health promotion and disease prevention strategies that can reduce childhood morbidity, promote healthy life styles for all children, and empower these children to become active, informed health consumers.

Major Health Problems of School-Age Children

Infectious Diseases

Before immunizations, many American children fell victim to epidemics of polio, diphtheria, pneumonia, measles, and pertussis. The majority of American children now receive adequate protection from these infectious diseases, but this protection does not reach some of the most vulnerable children—i.e., children of migrant farm workers (Lee, McDermott, and Elliott 1990) and children whose parents, in-

41

timidated by the costs of office visits and lost work time, delay immunizations until they are required for entrance to school (Igoe and Goodwin 1991). Pneumonia, meningitis, and influenza still contribute to the deaths of our nation's children and are the chief illness-related reasons for school absence (DHHS 1991) (see Table 5.1).

Environmental Hazards

Childhood asthma is increasing, especially among children who live in large metropolitan areas. Lead poisoning contributes significantly to developmental problems, and children who live in substandard housing are particularly at risk. America's schools—old and new—contain environmental hazards: asbestos, radon, and lead threaten students in older buildings while children attending some new schools encounter "sick-building syndrome" (Norback, Torgen, and Edling 1990). Violence in schools often renders the school psychological environment a veritable threat to children's well-being.

Unintentional Injuries

The leading cause of death in childhood—unintentional injuries—is also the most preventable. Nearly half of all childhood deaths are a result of unintentional injuries; half of these are caused by motor vehicle accidents. With the institution of automobile child-restraint laws, these rates have begun to decrease. Drownings and fire account for most other injury-related deaths, and injuries from falls and poisonings cause many non-fatal injuries among America's children.

Social and Economic Health Problems

Mental retardation, learning disorders, emotional and behavioral problems, vision and speech impairments, and homicide are more prevalent among children living in poverty than among those at higher socioeconomic levels (DHHS 1991). HIV infection and the effects of intrauterine cocaine exposure are the newest scourges affecting the health of the nation's children. Prenatal exposure to cocaine is associated with stillbirths, congenital malformations, premature births, intrauterine growth retardation, and hyperactivity (National Health/ Education Consortium 1991). Again, those children living in poverty are disproportionately affected. Dental caries and malnutrition are major, preventable health problems also affecting poor American children.

Nursing Interventions

The preventable nature of these major health concerns calls for nurses to intervene to improve the health of America's children. Public health nurses began focusing on child health at the beginning of this century

Table 5.1   Leading Age-Specific Health Problems of Children One Year to Twelve Years of Age

Leading Causes of Death	Common Health Problems	Anticipatory Guidance of Parents and Children
Pre-School Years		
Accidents	Developmental lag	• Injury prevention—seat belt and child restraint use; smoke detectors in homes, storage of firearms, drugs, toxic chemicals, matches/cigarette lighters out of reach and sight; playground safety rules and proper supervision.
Infections	Lead poisoning	
Child abuse	Infectious diseases	
		• Infectious disease prevention—immunizations; hygienic practices to control/prevent spread.
		• Child abuse prevention—crisis intervention availability: social support networks; counseling.
		• Lead poisoning prevention—environmental check; screening of high-risk children; teaching parents to recognize warning signs.
		• Developmental encouragement—regular well-child assessments; nutrition education; routine developmental screening; early referral.
School Years		
Accidents	Influenza and pneumonia	• Injury prevention—safety belts; smoke detectors in homes; proper storage of firearms, drugs, toxic chemicals, matches/cigarette lighters; bicycle safety helmets.
Congenital anomalies	Infections (ENT)	
Cancers, including leukemia	Malnutrition	
Homicide		• Promotion of healthy life style—diet and exercise; dental health; protection of skin against ultraviolet light.
Heart disease		• Prevention of infection—elimination of allergens and irritants from environments; prevention of spread of infection.
		• Prevention of malnutrition—identification of children at risk; nutrition education; monitoring of growth; referral of families to community food resources.

Adapted from Stanhope & Lancaster (1992) and DHHS (1991).

with the establishment of the Henry Street Settlement House in New York City tenements. Nearly 90 years later in the same city, a model outreach program has demonstrated the effectiveness of a nurse-run program in health care screening and health education for predominantly low-income children (Good and Berger 1989). Nurses have become advocates for the well-child health needs of chronically ill children and have developed models for public health nursing that address the health needs of all children.

In 1991, the ANA, Children's Action Network, American Academy of Pediatrics, and state nurses associations launched a media and public awareness campaign in major American cities to improve the immunization rate of the nation's children. This campaign included immunization events that offered screening, immunization assessments, actual immunizations, and information for follow-up (ANA 1991a). That same year, the University of Texas Medical Branch (Galveston) (1991) School of Nursing received funding from the Kellogg Foundation to develop a three-part health promotion program for use in community-based clinics. The program will develop bilingual video discs that provide families with information on nutrition during pregnancy, prevention of low birth-weight infants, immunization schedules, and guidelines on accident prevention among infants and toddlers.

Across the nation, nurses are responding to children's health needs, providing skilled nursing care in homes, health education and primary care in schools, disease prevention in community clinics, and health policy making in legislatures. The ultimate challenge is to reduce health disparities and achieve access to preventive services for all American children.

Child Development of Health Promotion

Childhood is the prime time for human development and the acquisition of knowledge and behaviors that will affect adult life. Current health education in American schools reflects this developmental perspective: most districts have anti-smoking education in elementary schools, along with alcohol and drug avoidance counseling; 24 percent of states require nutrition education through the 12th grade; and 50 percent of the states require comprehensive school health-education programs (DHHS 1991).

To be effective, health education must be developmentally appropriate. As children develop, their conceptions of health and illness reflect an increasing differentiation between the self and the world and between the mind and the body. Decision making skills, the basic prerequisite for the development of preventive health behavior, must be learned and used as children encounter choices about life style and health risk-taking behaviors during the formative years (see Table 5.2).

For example, children in the pre-operational level of cognitive development (ages three years to eight years) can be taught to identify independently many of their health needs, and to identify some realistic solutions. At the concrete operation cognitive level (ages eight years to ten years and older), children can learn to plan for and take the initiative to carry out most health care behaviors if they have learned trust and autonomy. They also can consider possible risks and benefits of health behaviors if they are allowed to participate in problem solving. Once formal operational cognitive skills are acquired (age 12 years and older), children can assume full responsibility for identifying health needs, determining possible solutions, and engaging in healthy behaviors (Foster, Hunsberger, and Anderson 1989).

Programs to Teach Children Health Promotion and Disease Prevention

A number of programs have been developed to encourage children's participation in their own health care. The National Fire Protection Association (1980) appealed to the developmental level of elementary children with its "Crawl on Your Belly Like GI Joe" burn prevention curriculum. Many large cities have developed programs that teach elementary school children violence prevention through conflict resolution. These programs are designed to change knowledge about and attitudes toward violence and to instill interpersonal skills for resolving conflicts nonviolently. HealthPACT (Igoe 1980) is a curriculum that teaches elementary school children to use five steps—Talk, Listen, Ask, Decide, Do (TLADD)—to become participatory health consumers. Not only do the children acquire essential skills, but their teachers, parents, and school nurses use TLADD as a guide when preparing children to assume responsibility for their own personal health habits. The TLADD skills are essential to children's learning about disease prevention and health promotion.

All effective pediatric health-promotion programs are based on understanding children's developing comprehension of time, the body, health, clinical procedures, illness, and death. Table 5.2 illustrates the developmental concepts that govern children's comprehension of the body, health, and illness.

Health Promotion, Health Protection, and Disease Prevention

For many years, nurses have taught concepts of health and disease prevention to relatively small, isolated groups of children. Recently, health promotion, health protection, and disease prevention have become

Table 5.2 Children's Comprehension of Time, the Body, Health, and Illness

Age/Cognitive Stage	Time	The Body	Health	Illness
Pre-operational thought (ages three years to eight years)	Beginning to distinguish today from yesterday and tomorrow, but understands the future as a "long time away." Begins to tell time.	Begins with no knowledge of internal body parts. Learns about location of major organs and some body processes.	Health involves a series of health practices. Health is apparent when one is able to perform usual activities.	Phenomenism and contagion are key concepts at this age. Perceives an external unrelated, concrete phenomenon as cause of illness. Perceives cause of illness as proximity between two events occurring by magic.
Concrete operational thought (ages eight years to ten years or older)	Understands time and events.	Learning concepts such as circulation and respiration. Enjoys excitement of learning.	Health is a sense of well-being evidenced by feeling good or being in shape.	Contamination and internalization are key concepts at this age. Perceives cause of illness as a person, object, or action external to the child that is harmful to the body. This stage evolves to perceiving illness as having an external cause that is located inside the body (getting a cold by breathing in air and germs).
Formal operational thought (age 12 years and older)	Beginning to identify self as part of the future, but may not be realistic about future goals.	As puberty begins, becomes anxious about body changes. Begins to understand concept of disease prevention.	Health is long-term physical, emotional/social stability; brief illness may cause temporary instability. Health is feeling good, in control of self, and able to participate in desired activities.	Physiologic and psychologic concepts are present. Perceives illness as malfunctioning or nonfunctioning organs or process. Begins to realize that psychologic actions and attitudes affect health and illness.

Adapted from Whaley and Wong (1989); Adams-Greenly (1991); and Foster, Hunsberger, and Anderson (1989).

popular topics and now are major national policy goals. *Healthy People 2000* (DHHS 1991) is the federal program committed to achieving three broad goals: 1) increase the span of healthy life for Americans, 2) reduce health disparities among Americans, and, 3) achieve access to preventive services for all Americans.

Health promotion activities relate to an individual's life style and are relevant to all age groups, including children. The *Healthy People 2000* health promotion priority areas focus on physical activity and fitness; nutrition; tobacco; alcohol and other drugs; family planning; mental health and mental disorders; violent and abusive behavior, and educational and community-based programs.

Health protection activities relate to environmental or regulatory measures designed to protect large population groups—for example, protecting children from the environmental hazards of tobacco smoke and lead. *Healthy People 2000* also identifies unintentional injuries, food and drug safety, and oral health as major areas of health protection activity for children.

Preventive health and preventive services include counseling, screening, immunization, or chemoprophylactic interventions for individuals in clinical settings. These activities include maternal and infant health, HIV infection, sexually transmitted diseases (STDs), immunization, and infectious disease prevention. In this category, school children are to receive age-appropriate HIV education beginning in the fourth grade (McGinnis and DeGraw 1991).

Meeting These Goals and Objectives

The challenge of the *Healthy People 2000* mandate is to combine scientific knowledge, professional skill, individual commitment, community support, and political will to enable people to achieve their potential to live full, active lives. Improving the health of American children requires a wide range of social and economic interventions. To achieve these broad goals of *Healthy People 2000*, age-related objectives have been developed. Some of the pediatric objectives are presented in Table 5.3.

ANA (1991b) has underscored this current commitment to the nation's health by introducing a new agenda for health care reform that calls for a basic core of essential health-care services. The basic components of this agenda include a restructured health system and a shift from the predominant focus on illness and cure to an orientation toward wellness and care. Specific action items include:

- provision and financing of a federally defined standard package of essential health-care services.
- a fiscally responsible phasing-in of essential services.

Table 5.3   Healthy People 2000 Objectives for Child Health

Objective	Services and Protection	Examples of Intervention
Physical Activity and Fitness Increase to at least 30 percent the proportion of people age six years and older who engage regularly in light to moderate physical activity for at least 30 minutes per day.	Increase to at least 50 percent the proportion of children in grades 1 through 12 who participate in daily physical education.	Increase the frequency of physical education classes for children in lower grades. Enroll more children in upper grades in physical education classes.
Nutrition Reduce dietary fat intake to an average of 30 percent of calories or less and average saturated fat intake to less than 10 percent of calories among people age two years and older.	Increase to at least 90 percent the proportion of school lunch and breakfast services that are consistent with current nutrition principles. Increase to at least 75 percent the proportion of America's schools that provide nutrition education.	School curriculum should help students develop behavioral skills to plan, prepare, and select healthful meals/snacks, with educational experiences provided in school cafeterias. School fund-raising activities that involve food (vending machines and concession stands) should reflect current nutrition principles.
Tobacco Reduce the initiation of cigarette smoking by children and youth so that no more than 15 percent become regular smokers by age 20 years.	Establish tobacco-free school environments. Include tobacco use prevention in curricula of all elementary schools.	Effective tobacco-use prevention programs emphasize the short-term consequences of tobacco use (decreased stamina, stained teeth, foul-smelling breath/clothes, and potential for addiction) and guided rehearsal of refusal skills.

Table 5.3   (continued)

Objective	Services and Protection	Examples of Intervention
Alcohol and Other Drugs		
Increase the proportion of high school seniors who perceive social disapproval associated with heavy use of alcohol, occasional use of marijuana, and experimentation with cocaine.	Provide to children in all school districts and private schools primary and secondary education programs in alcohol and other drugs.	Effective programs provide factual information about harmful effects of drugs, and support and strengthen students' resistance to using drugs. They collaborate with parents and other community members. Strong school policies, assessment, and referral for treatment and provision of support groups for drug users also are essential program components.
Immunization and Infectious Diseases		
Reduce indigenous cases of vaccine-preventable diseases among children to zero. Increase immunization levels to at least 95 percent for children in kindergarten through post-secondary educational institutions.	Expand immunization laws for schools to all states for all antigens. Improve the financing and delivery of immunizations for children and adults so that virtually no American faces a financial barrier to receiving recommended immunizations.	Target minority populations, as these groups appear to have substantially lower immunization levels than the general population.
Violent and Abusive Behavior		
Reduce homicides among children age three years and younger to no more than 3.1 per 100,000 people. Reduce to less than 25.2 per 1,000 children the rising incidence of maltreatment of children under age 18 years.	Extend protocols for routinely identifying, treating, and properly referring victims of child abuse to at least 90 percent of hospital ER departments. Extend to at least 45 states implementation of unexplained child-death review systems.	A pilot high-school curriculum teaches students about the magnitude of the violence problem, their vulnerability to violent injury, the role of anger in human interactions, and strategies for nonviolent forms of conflict resolution.

Adapted from: DHHS (1991); McGinnis and DeGraw (1991).

- planned change that will anticipate health services needs.
- planned reduction in health care costs.
- case management to reduce fragmentation of health care.
- provisions for long-term care.
- insurance reforms.
- increased access to services.

These national goals and objectives must be translated into services both for individual children and for the aggregate of school-age youth. Each individual child should have a primary care provider who performs appropriate health screening, treatment, and referral and who provides age-appropriate health counseling and health education. Nurses in public health, school health, community clinics, and primary care settings can develop programs to meet these identified health needs of the nation's children.

Schools are the logical setting in which to educate youngsters about health risks and health-promoting behaviors. An example is the health-promotion model program ("Heart Smart") for elementary school children created through collaboration between health professionals and educators (Downey, Greenberg, Virgilio, and Berensen 1989). School nurses who work with health educators can serve as a valuable resource to other nurses who want to undertake health promotion/disease prevention activities with children.

Successful health promotion and disease prevention programs follow these steps: 1) conduct needs assessments, 2) develop performance objectives, 3) use a variety of learning activities, 4) break course content into manageable sections, and, 5) evaluate the results (learning and behavior changes).

Nurses have always understood the importance of health promotion and disease prevention. The American public is just now beginning to appreciate nursing's role in children's health. Using the *Healthy People 2000* objectives and ANA's *Nursing's Agenda for Health Care Reform* as guidelines, nurses can capitalize on this heightened public awareness to develop new health promotion/disease prevention programs for the nation's children.

References

Adams-Greenly, M. 1991. Long-term survivors of childhood cancer: Psychosocial assessment and intervention at initial diagnosis. *Pediatrician* 8, 3–10.

American Nurses Association. 1991a. ANA to conduct child immunization program. *The American Nurse* 23, p. 3.

American Nurses Association. 1991b. *Nursing's agenda for health care reform.* Kansas City, MO: Author.

Downey, A.M., Greenberg, J.S., Virgilio, S.J., and Berenson, G.S. 1989. Health promotion model for "Heart Smart": The medical school, university, and community. *Health Values* 13, 31–46.

Foster, R., Hunsberger, M., and Anderson, J. 1989. *Family-centered nursing care of children.* Philadelphia: W.B. Saunders Co.

Good, J.M., and Berger, D.K. 1989. A model outreach program for health care screening. *J Pediatric Health Care* 3, 305–10.

Igoe, J.B. 1980. Project HealthPACT in action. *American Journal of Nursing* 80, 2016–2021.

Igoe, J.B., and Goodwin, L.D. 1991. Meeting the challenge of immunizing the nation's children. *Pediatric Nursing* 17, 590–593.

Lee, C.V., McDermott, S.W., and Elliott, C. 1990. The delayed immunization of children of migrant farm workers in South Carolina. *Public Health Reports* 105, 317–320.

McGinnis, J.M., and DeGraw, C. 1991. Healthy schools 2000: Creating partnerships for the decade. *Journal of School Health* 61, 292–332.

National Fire Protection Association. 1980. *Learn not to burn curriculum: A fire prevention and safety education program for school children* (3rd ed.). Quincy, MA: Battery March Park.

National Health/Education Consortium. 1991. The relationship of health to learning: Healthy brain development. Washington, DC: Author.

Norback, D., Torgen, M., and Edling, D. 1990. Volatile organic compounds, respirable dust, and personal factors related to prevalence and incidence of sick building syndrome in primary schools. *British Journal of Industrial Medicine* 47, 733–741.

Stanhope, M., and Lancaster, J. 1992. *Community health nursing.* St. Louis: Mosby-Year Book.

University of Texas Medical Branch News and Information Office. 1991. UTMB School of Nursing receives $1.3 million Kellogg grant for community health education. Galveston, TX: Author.

U.S. Department of Health and Human Services, Public Health Service. 1991. *Healthy People 2000.* DHHS Publication No. (PHS) 91-50213. Washington, DC: US Government Printing Office.

Whaley, L.F., and Wong, D.L. 1989. *Essentials of pediatric nursing* (3rd ed.). St. Louis: C.V. Mosby.

6

Prevention: Adolescent Health

Ann L. O'Sullivan, Ph.D., R.N., F.A.A.N.
Associate Professor
School of Nursing
University of Pennsylvania

and

Theresa Apriceno-Tesoro, R.N., M.S.N., C.S., P.N.P.
Lecturer
School of Nursing
University of Pennsylvania

Adolescence is a challenging period for both the adolescent and his or her family, friends, and community. The major task facing the individual during this period is to develop a set of healthy behaviors. Many authors attest to the fact that younger teens have more difficulty than do older adolescents in engaging in positive health behaviors, whether it is body building, safe sex, or managing their anger. The degree to which adolescents succeed in establishing healthy behavior is associated with several factors including parental, peer, cognitive, emotional, and environmental influences.

Because categorization often lends clarity to a complex issue, adolescent health is discussed in this chapter in terms of physical health, mental health, and sexual health.

Physical Health

Oral Health

The number of dental cavities is much higher among adolescents than young children. Toothbrushing is an essential daily activity, and a new toothbrush should be used every three months. Because two-thirds of tooth decay occurs only on the chewing surfaces, adolescents should receive protective sealants on the chewing surfaces of permanent second molars.

Nutrition

Obese adolescents experience psychological stress and their obesity may persist into adulthood. Eating disorders such as anorexia and bulimia surface at this time because of our society's over-emphasis on thinness.

Calcium is important for the formation of bones, and iron is important for women of childbearing age to prevent iron-deficiency anemia. Adolescents must read food labels to make sure they eat three or more servings rich in calcium and know how to obtain iron-rich foods when needed. At least one quart of water per day is important for all.

Exercise

All adolescents need physical activity promoting cardiorespiratory fitness three or more days per week, for at least twenty minutes each time. Physical activities that promote cardiorespiratory fitness include brisk walking, stair climbing, dancing, jogging or running, lap swimming, rope jumping, rowing, racquet sports, and competitive group sports. Weight lifting with few repetitions will neither promote cardiorespiratory fitness nor maintain muscular strength, muscular endurance, or flexibility.

Risk of Unintentional Injuries

Motor-vehicle accident deaths among youth ages 15 years through 24 years occur at the rate of 36.9 per 100,000 people. The year 2000 objective is to lower the rate to 33 per 100,000 people. This reduction can only occur with continued reductions in drunk driving, increased use of seat belts and mass transit; and improvement of pedestrian, motorcycle, and bicycle safety. Increased use of helmets by motorcyclists and bicyclists is essential; presently only 60 percent of motorcyclists and 10 percent of bicyclists use helmets.

Lowering the volume of stereos and headphones may also prevent problems of eventual hearing loss. A good rule to follow is: If you start to hear buzzing, the sound is damaging your ears.

Violence

Homicide is the number-one cause of death among African-American adolescents, and the second leading cause of death among all adolescents. Most homicides are a result of use of a firearm during an argument between people who know one another. Using firearms and knives is most often what turns a violent fight into a lethal event. Between 2 percent and 14 percent of eighth graders carry knives to school daily. Other reports indicate that 135,000 youth bring guns to school each day.

Physical fighting results in hundreds of homicides and uncounted numbers of non-fatal injuries among adolescents, which result in loss of school and work days. Teaching and reviewing conflict resolution skills with adolescents may decrease their risk of becoming victims or perpetrators of violence.

Tobacco, Alcohol, and Other Drugs

The "gateway" concept suggests that experimentation with drugs usually begins with cigarettes, alcohol, or marijuana, and then progresses to other, more dangerous mind-altering or addictive substances like cocaine, LSD, or amphetamines. Most people start smoking during adolescence, with experimentation beginning at a much younger age.

Studies have shown that it is easier to prevent the initiation of smoking than it is to sustain an intervention that helps an adolescent quit smoking. Most users of moist or dry snuff and chewing tobacco are teenage boys. All smokeless tobacco products contain nicotine and their use may lead to cigarette smoking.

Alcohol-related motor vehicle accidents are the leading cause of death and spinal cord injuries among adolescents. Surveys have defined heavy drinking by youth as five or more drinks on one occasion. Now that the legal drinking age has been raised to twenty-one in all states, parents and all other adults must foster stricter enforcement of the minimum age laws. Perceived risk of psychological or physical harm and social disapproval have decreased the use of marijuana and cocaine among adolescents. Radio and television advertising needs to use these prevention factors to decrease the use of cigarettes and alcohol.

Screening for tobacco, alcohol, or drug use is essential to establish the existence of predisposing risk factors, problems in major life areas, and peer use and personal use characteristics. One can obtain accurate data asking validated screening questions using an organizing acronym, e.g., *CAGE*. A good lead-in question could be: "Have you ever been concerned about your (or someone else's) use of alcohol, tobacco, or other drugs?" followed by:

- Have you ever felt the need to **C**ut down on drinking, smoking, or drug use?
- Have you ever felt **A**nnoyed by criticism about your drinking, smoking, or drug use?
- Have you ever felt **G**uilty about your drinking, smoking, or drug use?
- Have you ever felt **G**uilty about something you said or did while you were drinking, smoking, or using drugs?
- Have you ever taken a morning **E**ye-opener?

Minor Common Illnesses

For young adolescents (ages 11 years to 14 years) and older adolescents (ages 15 years to 20 years), routine physical examinations and symptoms of a throat problem are in the top three reasons for a physician office visit. Routine prenatal examination was the principal reason for girls in the older group, and acne and pimples or a skin rash make up one of the top four reasons for a visit by any adolescent.

Serious Chronic Illness

Asthma affects approximately 10 million Americans. The death rate from asthma among African-Americans is three times as high as the rate among white people, although the two groups contract asthma at the same rate. Awareness, for an adolescent, of the individual triggers of an asthma attack and how to use his or her medicines may prevent serious episodes. In addition to taking precautions against asthma, most adolescents need booster dT, a second MMR immunization, and the three-shot series of Hepatitis B vaccine.

Mental Health

High levels of stress or conflict at home, along with physical, sexual, or emotional abuse, often contribute to depression and other psychological difficulties for adolescents. According to Congress' Office of Technology Assessment (1991), 12 percent of American youth need some type of mental health service but fewer than one in eight actually secures any treatment.

School attendance is a major indicator of mental health. Dropout rates in the United States indicate that 12.6 percent of 16- to 24-year-olds have not completed high school. Adolescents drop out of school for many reasons including boredom; academic failure; mental, physical, or sexual health problems; and family and financial problems. In some parts of our country, more than 50 percent of freshmen who enter high school never graduate.

Suicide

Suicide among youths ages 15 years to 19 years is on a steady increase and was the second leading cause of death in this age group by 1987. Contributing factors include previous suicide attempts, inadequate treatment, precipitous life events, substance abuse, family history of suicide or psychiatric disorders, exposure to suicidal behavior, family violence, and availability of guns in the home. Unlike suicides in adults that occur with depression, suicides in teenagers tend to be impulsive acts that may not be related to depression.

General guidelines for the assessment of an adolescent who has attempted suicide include:

- Take all suicide threats seriously. Do not make a distinction between attempts and gestures.
- Proceed with a calm, supportive, non-judgmental attitude.
- Interview the adolescent (preferably within the first 24 hours) and family members or group home staff, both separately and together.
- Listen patiently. Use open-ended questions and allow time for responses.
- Be direct and specific whenever responses are unclear, contradictory, or confusing.
- Document information thoroughly.
- Explain the process of assessment and management.
- Reinforce the danger of suicidality with adolescent and family or group home staff.
- Provide continuity and support to the adolescent and family throughout any hospitalization.

Assessment Instruments for Mental Health Issues

The following self-report instruments may be helpful in assessing depression and coping responses.

- Beck Depression Inventory (eighth-grade reading level, twenty-one items) or Kovacs Depression Inventory (Kovacs 1985) (first-grade reading level, 23 items).
- A-COPE (Adolescent Coping Orientation for Problem Experiences) (Patterson et al. 1983) (54-item coping inventory designed to identify the behaviors adolescents find helpful in managing problems or difficult situations).

Parents may want to believe that their child or adolescent will simply outgrow a mental or behavioral problem, but recent research suggests that untreated depression in early adolescence often leads to chronic difficulties in teenage years—especially in girls—and to adult depression. Anxiety disorders, first diagnosed around age 15 years, persist through adolescence and into adulthood if untreated.

Sexual Health

Sexual Development

To assess timely sexual development of the adolescent throughout puberty, correctly assigning sexual maturation states needs to occur at each visit. For boys, this means rating the genitalia and pubic hair. A boy should reach genitals SMR (sexual maturation ratio) 2 by 13.7 years or pubic hair SMR 2 by 15.1 years. In girls, the breasts and pubic hair are classified and concern should occur if a female is not menstruating by 16 years.

Sexual Activity

Adolescents face constant pressures about sexual intercourse, most significantly from peers. *Healthy People 2000* estimates that, currently, 27 percent of girls and 33 percent of boys have engaged in intercourse by age 15 years. This number doubles by age 17 years, when 50 percent of girls and 66 percent of boys report having had sexual intercourse.

Accurate information about the consequences of intercourse—pregnancy, STDs, AIDS—needs to be given nonjudgmentally. Information about abstinence and support needs to be provided as well. Role playing can help the adolescent work through dating and social situations before problems occur, and does not require training. Support for the teen's decision must be available.

Contraception

When any adolescent—male or female—is engaging in sexual intercourse or is considering it, contraception needs to be discussed. Most adolescents seek contraceptive health care about one year after initiating sexual intercourse. According to *Healthy People 2000*, 63 percent of adolescents ages 15 years to 19 years reported using a contraceptive method at first intercourse. The condom was the most reported method; only 2 percent used oral contraceptive pills. Unfortunately, because of condoms' sporadic use and lack of effectiveness, many adolescents become pregnant within six months of initiating intercourse.

All adolescents should be encouraged to use condoms with an additional effective method of birth control. In 1988, only 26 percent of unmarried young women reported that their partner used a condom at last intercourse. Stressing the fact that more adolescents are using condoms will help the adolescent overcome fears of not conforming to their peer group. It also is helpful to rehearse with a teen how to ask someone to use a condom or any birth control method.

All teens should be aware of the accessibility of over-the-counter methods of birth control, such as a sponge and spermacides (teens prefer a suppository or pre-packaged foam because they are compact and easy to conceal and use). A new form of spermicide, the *vaginal contraceptive film* (VCF), should also gain popularity with teens for the same reasons. It is a thin, two-inch square containing nonoxynol-9 which dissolves.

The diaphragm as a birth control method seems to be chosen only by highly motivated and well-educated adolescent girls. Oral contraceptive pills are better accepted and far more effective at preventing pregnancy. The major obstacle to their effectiveness is that adolescents stop taking the pill for various reasons while continuing to engage in intercourse. Diligent follow-up on missed appointments or directly asking when the last pill was taken will help identify teens who have stopped taking pills.

Norplant and Depo-Provera can provide the adolescent with a highly effective contraceptive method which requires little intervention by the teen. Depo-Provera, a synthetic progesterone, protects against pregnancy for three months after a single injection. The need for injections four times a year may adversely affect compliance in adolescents. We have found a growing acceptance for Norplant, the subdermal progesterone that is effective for five years. Diligently monitoring and screening teens on Norplant for STDs is important.

Maintaining Fertility and Preventing Disease

By the age of 21 years, approximately 25 percent of sexually active young adults will have had a STD. The consequences of some of these infections are decreased fertility or death. For women, *pelvic inflammatory disease* (PID) can cause chronic pelvic pain, dyspareunia, ectopic pregnancy, and infertility. It is estimated that one in seven women of reproductive age has had PID, with the highest rates occurring among adolescents. Because it is difficult to convince an adolescent that putting off intercourse or limiting the number of sexual partners may benefit him or her later in life, frequent screening of sexually active adolescents for diseases and conducting routine PAP smears for girls are imperative.

Unfortunately, STDs occur more commonly in adolescents. For men, the highest rate of gonorrhea occurs in 15- to 24-year-olds. Over the past decade, the number of adolescents acquiring syphilis has risen, a worrisome trend. *Human papillomavirus* (HPV) infection rates have been reported to be as high as 38 percent to 46 percent for adolescent and young women. HPV can result in infections of the cervix, epithelial cell changes on PAP smear, and low-grade cervical intraepithelial neoplasia.

The Centers for Disease Control (CDC) reported in 1990 that only 3.8 percent of AIDS cases occurred in the 13- to 19-year age group. However, there is an eight- to ten-year incubation period, so a significant proportion of the 20 percent of the 20- to 29-year-olds with AIDS acquired the HIV virus in their adolescence. Furthermore, heterosexual transmission of the disease in this age group has increased. Women comprise 20 percent of adolescents with AIDS, whereas only 9 percent of the adults are women. Unfortunately, adolescents are not getting the message about safe sex.

Adverse Sexual Experiences

Unwanted sexual encounters can vary from an unwanted touch to rape. They can involve a family member, an acquaintance, or a stranger. They happen to males and females and have long-term emotional consequences. Health surveys estimate that 7 percent to 15 percent of older adolescents report at least one episode of involuntary sexual intercourse, and that girls are more likely to report such experiences than boys. Approximately half of all non-voluntary sexual experiences occur before the age of 14 years.

Pregnancy

Of the developed countries, the United States has one of the highest adolescent pregnancy rates, despite the fact that in most of the other developed countries there are more adolescents engaging in sexual intercourse. The rates for unintentional pregnancy in our country are 50 percent to 85 percent higher than those in Europe. Rates of abortion are about the same. Adolescents delay early detection of pregnancy, sometimes limiting their choice of options, delaying onset of prenatal care, and undergoing more risky second-trimester abortions.

Keys to Communication

If a health care provider appears distant, aloof, or rushed, the adolescent will not talk about what is on his or her mind. Other times, the adolescent is too shy or uncomfortable with his or her body to raise sensitive but important health concerns such as drug use or STDs. Health education could help adolescents overcome feelings of fear, embarrassment, or denial that, "It couldn't happen to me." The most important way to promote open communication between provider and adolescent client is to ensure confidentiality. Providers who cannot should refer the adolescent to a program where confidentiality can be guaranteed.

Screening questions using a mnemonic device (e.g., "HEADS") can help organize data collection during any interview. HEADS stands for Home, Education, Activities/Affect, Drugs, and Sex:

- **H**ome. Who lives in your house with you? When there is stress or tension, what is it usually about? Whom does it usually involve?
- **E**ducation. What are you good at in school? What is hard for you? How do your grades compare to last year's grades? Has anyone been concerned about your school performance?
- **A**ctivities/Affect. What do you do for fun? What do you do with friends? What do you do with your free time? Do you find yourself getting into trouble more now than before? What kinds of things usually get you into trouble?
- **D**rugs. Use CAGE questions listed earlier (see p. 55).
- **S**ex. Most young people become interested in relationships at your age. Have you ever had a sexual relationship with anyone?

If a teen knows that you care, you can ask any question.

References

American Medical Association. 1990. *Healthy youth 2000—National health promotion and disease prevention objectives for adolescents.* Chicago: Author.

Gans, J.E., Blyth, D.A., Ister, A.B., and Gaveras, L.L. 1990. *American adolescents: How healthy are they?* Chicago: American Medical Association.

Gans, J.E., McManus, M.A., and Newacheck, P.W. 1991. *Adolescent health care: Use, costs, and problems of access.* Chicago: American Medical Association.

Institute of Medicine. 1989. *Research on children and adolescents with mental, behavioral, and developmental disorders: Mobilizing a national initiative.* Washington, DC: National Academy Press.

Kovacs, M. 1985. The children's depression inventory (CDI). *Psychopharmacological Bulletin* 21, 995–998,

Patterson, J.M., and McCubbin, H.I. 1983. *Adolescent-coping orientation for problem experiences.* Madison, WI.: Family Stress Coping and Health Project.

U.S. Congress, Office of Technology Assessment. 1991. *Adolescent health—Volume I: Summary and policy options.* Washington, DC: U.S. Government Printing Office.

7

Prevention: Adults with Chronic Disease

Carol L. Macnee, Ph.D., R.N.
Associate Professor of Family-Community Nursing
East Tennessee State University
Johnson City, TN

and

Jean Goeppinger, Ph.D., R.N., F.A.A.N.
Professor and Chair
Department of Community and Mental Health Nursing
School of Nursing
University of North Carolina
Chapel Hill, NC

Planning preventive care for adults who have chronic diseases requires thinking about prevention from a unique perspective. Traditional primary and secondary prevention activities focus on preventing disease and promoting its early detection in order to cure it. Frequently, these activities occur in childhood—e.g., immunizations and vision and hearing screening. Even tertiary prevention, although generally targeted at adults, is traditionally described as beginning early in the period of *recovery* from illness in order to optimize the effects of treatment and to prevent complications (Pender 1987).

Yet, chronic diseases—specifically, cardiovascular disease, cancer, and cerebrovascular disease—are the top three causes of illness and death in adults 40 years old and older in the United States, and, by definition, chronic diseases have neither cure nor full recovery. Chronic diseases are further differentiated from acute illnesses because they are often related to health behaviors and life styles, as opposed to specific etiologic agents, and they often have an insidious onset and endure over a long and indefinite period. Therefore, the focus of prevention in adults with chronic diseases must be shifted away from cure and toward a focus on quality of life and promoting optimal functioning.

This chapter discusses prevention for adults with arthritis. The chronic disease of arthritis was chosen as an example because it is the second most prevalent and commonly reported chronic condition for people of all ages, second only to chronic sinusitis. The overall prevalence rate of arthritis is 130 per 1,000 people; 18.8 percent of people who have activity limitations in the United States report that arthritis is the primary source of those limitations (DeVellis, Gerber, and Wilson 1991). Arthritis is, in fact, the chronic disease most likely to cause disability. Like all chronic diseases, arthritis has no cure and although health care professionals provide care for persons with arthritis through periodic evaluations, individuals with arthritis must assume responsibility for a lifetime of self-care for the condition and its effects on their functioning.

Prevention of Disability in Chronic Disease

Preventive care for adults with chronic diseases requires thinking about prevention of dysfunction or disability due to a disease process, rather than prevention of the disease itself. An image often used to describe public health care is that of bodies floating down a fast-flowing river; the river represents illness and the bodies portray people affected by it. Medical care is often described as a "downstream endeavor" because the treatment of illness is similar to pulling bodies out of the river one by one as they float down (Butterfield 1990). Public health is considered an "upstream endeavor," focusing on preventing whatever factors in the environment (physical, social, political, or economic) are pushing people into the river to begin with.

This same image can be used when thinking about prevention for people with chronic diseases, only the river now represents disability and dysfunction. Rather than focusing on treatment and rehabilitation of individuals who are disabled and have decreased levels of functioning (pulling the bodies out downstream), nurses need to "look upstream" to what is causing individuals with chronic diseases to become disabled (Butterfield 1990).

To identify preventive activities for people with chronic diseases—activities that will, for example, prevent disability—it is helpful to consider WHO's classification of impairments, disabilities, and handicaps. This classification describes four progressive levels of disease consequences starting with the disease itself and progressing to impairment, disability, and handicap (see Figure 7.1).

At the first, or disease, level, something abnormal occurs within the individual. In arthritis, the disease level would be the inflammation and possibly beginning erosion of selected joints. Traditional primary prevention is aimed at preventing this level from occurring. Current knowledge about the causes of most types of arthritis is insufficient to support primary prevention. This is not the case, however, with cardiovascular disease and many forms of cancer.

Fig. 7.1. The World Health Organization's Classification of
Impairments, Disabilities, and Handicaps

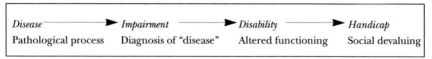

Disease ——————▶	*Impairment* —————▶	*Disability* —————▶	*Handicap*
Pathological process	Diagnosis of "disease"	Altered functioning	Social devaluing

Impairment is the second level of disease consequences. At this
level, the individual becomes aware and recognizes that something is
wrong. This is the point at which clinical disease usually is diagnosed
and medical treatment begins. Individuals with arthritis at the level of
impairment know that they have been experiencing pain or stiffness
because they have arthritis. Traditional secondary prevention targets
early treatment at the impairment level.

The third and fourth levels of disease consequences identify the
areas for prevention that are unique to people with chronic diseases.
The third level is disability, the point at which individuals' functioning
is altered as a result of their impairments. This altered functioning
may be behavioral, cognitive, or psychological. Individuals with arthritis may experience disability as a decreased ability to perform their
jobs, daily routines, and social activities, and may experience feelings
of discouragement or helplessness. At the fourth level of disease consequences, the handicap level, individuals' altered functioning or disabilities put them at a relative disadvantage to others. They are viewed as
functioning differently from other people and therefore as being
somehow less capable than others. For example, individuals with
arthritis at the handicapped level may be perceived as incapable of
working steadily outside or within the home, or unable to provide certain types of self-care.

Whereas traditional tertiary prevention is targeted at preventing disabilities, as well as promoting recovery from illness, it is more helpful
to think about *prevention for individuals with chronic disease as prevention
of progression from one level of disease consequences to another* (see Figure
7.2). Thus, primary and secondary prevention for individuals with
chronic diseases is aimed at keeping impairments from becoming disabilities and targeting early changes in function secondary to impairments so that they may be modified. Tertiary prevention is concerned
with preventing disabilities from becoming handicaps.

For example, primary prevention for an individual with arthritis
would be aimed at preventing the pain and stiffness of the disease
from negatively affecting the individual's job performance, social life,
household tasks, and personal care. This might be done through education about use of heat and cold, exercise, and medication to control

Fig. 7.2. Points for Prevention in the WHO Classification of Levels of Impairments, Disability, Handicaps

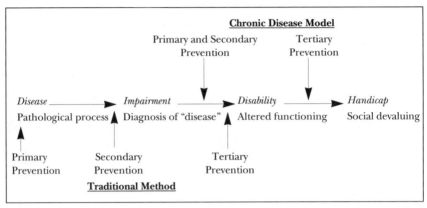

symptoms. In addition, modifications in the pacing and sequence of daily activities and the use of selected assistive devices for joint protection would promote prevention of disability. Primary prevention might also include participation in a self-help group to provide emotional and social support and role models of optimal functioning. Thus, primary prevention for individuals with impairment from a chronic disease would emphasize keeping the individual "out of the river" of disability.

Secondary prevention of disability for individuals with arthritis might include early recognition that changes in ability to function at work or at home require problem solving. For an individual employed in a physically strenuous occupation, for instance, secondary prevention might include retraining to allow a position or job change. For the homemaker, secondary prevention might involve reorganizing the household to decrease or eliminate the need to climb stairs. In either case, the goal is the early modification of personal and environmental factors that limit the individual's functioning in order to prevent loss of function or disability. These interventions would also keep individuals "high and dry."

DeVellis, Gerber, and Wilson (1991) stressed the altered focus needed when considering prevention of arthritis disability. They provided an excellent and detailed description of strategies at the primary, secondary, and tertiary levels for each of the six major categories of rheumatic disease. However, in their categorization of prevention strategies, they tended to take a more traditional view of prevention. Therefore, many of the strategies listed as tertiary prevention could also be viewed as preventing movement from impairment to disability levels within the WHO classification, hence, representing a form of primary and secondary prevention.

Although this chapter focuses on prevention related to chronic disease experienced by adults, the individual with a chronic disease still has traditional primary and secondary prevention needs in areas unaffected by the chronic disease. Thus, women with arthritis are no more or less at risk for breast cancer than are other women, and they need education and encouragement to receive regular screening (secondary prevention). Similarly, traditional primary prevention focused on eating low-fat foods is just as important for the individual with arthritis as it is for anyone else. In fact, recognizing and stressing to the client the relationships between selected "treatments" focused on their chronic disease (such as weight loss to decrease joint strain) and promoting their health in general, may facilitate a more positive outlook about these self-care activities.

Prevention of Handicap from Disability

Despite efforts at prevention of disability subsequent to impairment, over time, individuals with chronic diseases often experience diminished functioning. "Upstream efforts," however, can prevent a disability from becoming a handicap for many of these individuals. Prevention of handicaps can be thought of as tertiary prevention.

Most of the prevention strategies discussed so far could be seen as focusing only on the individual with a chronic disease. But many of the strategies just suggested also require intervention at the level of the family or the community. For example, reorganizing a household so the homemaker does not have to climb stairs would likely involve all family members in planning and implementation (e.g., moving a laundry area to the main floor or changing a first-floor study into a bedroom). Similarly, primary prevention through participation in a support group might well require the nurse to help form such a group, a community-wide intervention.

Therefore, prevention of disabilities from impairments requires care focused on the individual, the family, and the community. Interventions to prevent disabilities from becoming handicaps have an even greater focus on family and community levels of care, because handicaps reflect society's view of the individual, not just the individual's personal perceptions. In order to be viewed and to view oneself as disadvantaged relative to others, family and community members must somehow respond to the individual in ways that emphasize that disadvantage. Our society reveres youth, health, and vitality, for example, so the individual who has altered physical or psychological functioning is viewed as somehow disadvantaged.

Given the societal response to individuals with disabilities, tertiary prevention of handicaps from disability requires that the nurse challenge existing social structures in order to promote alternate views and opportunities. Stevens (1989) suggested that radical reconceptualization of the environment provides a useful approach to challenging social structures.

Critical social theory uses the processes of critique, dialogue, "conscientization," and action to change existing power structures and systems. Thus, a critical examination of social responses to individuals with different abilities—e.g., to individuals with arthritis experiencing altered ability to ambulate or carry out fine motor activities—may reveal that building designs and city plans discount the value of these individuals. By not considering how a differently abled person might access a store, bank, school, or office building, society sends a clear message that he or she does not matter.

The process of mutual dialogue among architects, nurses, persons who are differently abled, city planners, business people, and others about the impact of physical barriers on access to buildings can clarify and raise the consciousness of people within a community about their implicit assumptions. The process of conscientization can in turn lead to action to promote social change so that those with different functioning are not viewed as less able than others. In the example of inaccessible buildings, actions might be to support a citywide code that all public buildings must be wheelchair-accessible and have punch-bar doors, or to adopt monitoring mechanisms to ensure that new construction is in compliance with state and federal guidelines for barrier-free public buildings. Interventions at the tertiary level to prevent handicaps could use critical social theory to inform community and societal changes.

Although interventions to promote social change are basic to the tertiary prevention of handicaps, interventions to promote a sense of control and positive worth in individuals with disabilities are also strategies for prevention of handicaps. Goeppinger, Arthur, Baglioni, Brunk, and Brunner (1989) developed an arthritis self-care education program based on the theory of learned helplessness. The program suggests that when individuals do not see a connection between their actions and desired outcomes, they develop feelings of helplessness and depression. Because arthritis is often unpredictable and inconsistent, individuals with arthritis are at particular risk for seeing themselves as helpless in the face of their disease, and, hence, less able than others, or handicapped. Interventions that focus on promoting a sense of control over symptom management (versus symptom expression) and self-worth in individuals with disabilities can both prevent development of handicaps and potentially modify or decrease the extent to which an individual is handicapped.

The self-care education program presented by Goeppinger et al. (1989), "Bone Up on Arthritis," stresses how individuals can control the way they respond to their arthritis, and has been shown to lead to decreased feelings of helplessness in persons with arthritis. Decreases in helpless feelings have, in turn, been shown to explain decreases in pain. Strategies used to promote a sense of control include relaxation and problem-solving techniques, as well as the use of exercise, rest, and medications. The program is community-based and utilizes trained community residents as facilitators or leaders of small groups. A program developed from a related theory of perceived control—self-efficacy theory—has been tested and found to be effective as well (Lorig, Shoor, and Holman 1985).

Conclusion

Many individuals over the age of 40 years have one or more chronic diseases, and nurses need to take an active role in preventive care for these individuals. Prevention for individuals with chronic diseases requires a focus on promoting maximal functioning and enhanced quality of life, rather than preventing acute illness. Specific strategies, such as balanced use of exercise and rest, are appropriate interventions to prevent progression of impairment to disability or handicap. Key to successful prevention for adults with chronic diseases is the development of an understanding of the process of prevention. This understanding includes recognizing key points in the progression of the consequences of disease, where looking upstream can prevent more bodies from falling into the river of disability and handicap. Interventions can be primary, secondary, and tertiary; aimed at the individual, the family, the community, or society; and focused on promoting individual control and social change.

References

Berg, R.L., and Cassells, J.S., eds. 1990. *The second fifty years: Promoting health and preventing disability.* Washington, DC: Institute of Medicine, National Academy Press.

Butterfield, P.G. 1990. Thinking upstream: Nurturing a conceptual understanding of the societal context of health behavior. *Advances in Nursing Science* 12(2), 1–8.

DeVellis, R.F., Gerber, L.H., and Wilson, M.G. 1991. Prevention of arthritis disability. Conference on Biopsychosocial Contributions to the Management of Arthritis Disability. St. Louis.

Goeppinger, J., Arthur, M.W., Baglioni, A.J., Brunk, S.E., and Brunner, C.M. 1989. A reexamination of the effectiveness of self-care education for persons with arthritis. *Arthritis and Rheumatism* 32(6), 706–716.

Lorig, K., Shoor, S., and Holman, H.R. 1985. Experimental evidence that changes in psychological factors are associated with changes in arthritis pain. *Arthritis and Rheumatism* 28(suppl), p. S29.

Pender, N.J. 1987. *Health promotion in nursing practice* (2nd ed.). Norwalk, CT: Appleton & Lange.

Stevens, P.E. 1989. A critical social reconceptualization of environment in nursing: Implications for methodology. *Advances in Nursing Science* 11(4), 56–68.

8

Prevention: Work Site Wellness

John Fehir, Ph.D., R.N., C.
Evaluation Consultant
De Madres a Madres
Houston, TX

A rare opportunity will present itself to America's health professionals in the next few years. Disease prevention and health promotion interventions can be offered to and influence more than 210 million people through the nation's work sites. Community, public, and occupational health nurses must seize this opportunity to intervene directly at the work site with the nation's 100 million workers, most of whom live with at least one other person who will be indirectly affected.

Most working, middle-age adults are relatively healthy, do not need disease care, and have few reasons to contact a health care professional. Thus, very few opportunities exist for nurses to interact with people of this age group. The work site constitutes an efficient, unique opportunity for nurses to prevent disease, teach and guide, and motivate people to promote their own health and wellness. Nursing is the health care force that can effectively interact with workers and their families to help them shape their own health and wellness.

Although nurses are justifiably concerned about disease prevention, it is becoming increasingly important in our society for nurses to intervene at new levels of health promotion to enhance wellness long before disease becomes evident. Disease prevention and health promotion should be initiated while people are at work. Now more than ever before, there are many reasons why work site wellness is important.

Most of the employed people in the United States are under the age of 65 years and are at the greatest risk for premature morbidity and mortality in spite of being, overall, a healthy group. Preventive and health promotion interventions completed at the work site help reduce the burgeoning amount and rate of increase of national health care expenditures, delay the onset of costly chronic diseases, reduce the need for expensive disease care before old age, prolong quality longevity, and shorten the time of costly terminal events.

Health Care Costs

There are at least two types of measurable costs that indicate effectiveness of work-site disease prevention and health promotion programs: the costs of risks and cost savings. The cost of risks such as alcohol and drug abuse, injury, obesity, smoking, and stress are well documented and are reason for concern and action by the Secretary of Health and Human Services (DHHS 1991).

High-risk employees have significantly higher health care costs and absenteeism due to illness than do low-risk employees. For example, employees who smoke a pack of cigarettes per day have 18 percent higher medical claim costs than those of people who do not smoke (Jose and Anderson 1991).

The results of disease prevention and health promotion programs are reflected in *cost savings* for both employers and workers. After workers have the benefit of nurse intervention to promote their health and the cost of such intervention is accounted for, the amount of money not spent on health care can be measured. For example, for 15,267 high-risk employees, after six years of intervention, annual savings in health care claims alone were $1.8 million; for 40-year-old employees who reduced several risks, health-care claims savings were $8,966 per person per year (Jose and Anderson 1991).

People desire more than ever to be happy, healthy, and satisfied with their lives, and to enhance the quality of their lives. Health promotion addresses each of these goals.

Nursing Goals

Work-site nurses are concerned with traditional nursing goals such as monitoring health, providing emergency and temporary care, and teaching about preventing work-site injuries. More importantly, these nurses are increasingly involved in case management practices that are not only cost-efficient but result in disease prevention and improved total health and wellness. Case management is an ideal practice modality for prevention and health promotion because it allows a comprehensive, one-on-one health-care delivery approach that is family-centered and interdisciplinary.

Work sites are becoming the focus of efforts to initiate, adopt, and maintain healthy life style behaviors. Work-site nurses facilitate a host of programs designed to allow these life style behaviors to change and thus usher in a new and better method of health care delivery. Some examples of these programs are:

- alcohol and tobacco use cessation
- exercising as a lifelong habit
- stress management
- better nutrition and eating habits
- personal and family growth and development.

To deliver health care, work-site nurses will serve more frequently as consultants to small work groups of less than 50 employees. All of these efforts complement and reflect the goals of ANA. Following are some objectives pertaining to health care at the work site.

- The health care delivery system must change and incorporate a mix of public and private plans and resources, including those of the work site.
- Health care delivery must be refocused to seek a balance between prevention and cure. It is far more costly to provide health care after illness strikes than to prevent disease in the first place.
- Every person is entitled to a core of essential health care services, most of which can be delivered at the work site.
- Better access to health care is mandatory and the work site can facilitate this goal.

Employer Goals

In our competitive international trade market, it has become economically prudent for employers to have healthy, satisfied workers because they generally are more productive and efficient. Employers are vitally interested in workers' health because health status and costs are directly linked to productivity and profitability (Johnson 1991). For these reasons, many major U.S. companies, including Tenneco, Hershey Foods, Mesa Oil, U-Haul, Adolf Coors, Foldcraft, and Baker-Hughes have various types of health promotion programs—some with and some without incentives—for their employees. By 1995, half of all major U.S. companies will offer some type of incentive for their employees to practice health-promoting life style behaviors.

The Secretary of Health and Human Services has challenged U.S. health professionals to use the work site as a base for disease prevention and health promotion interventions (DHHS 1991). In addition to a specific set of fifteen objectives directed toward occupational safety and health, *Healthy People 2000: National Health Promotion and Disease Prevention Objectives* specifies 33 other work-related objectives designed to increase workers' health, safety, and wellness as well as decrease incidences of accidents and illness.

Nursing Action

The ANA and the American Association of Occupational Health Nurses (AAOHN) work at the local, state, and national levels to monitor and promote worker health and safety. Regular meetings with politicians and federal agency staff—during which examples of nurses' cost-effective primary health care at the work site is provided to government representatives—are a continuous priority for AAOHN leaders. Continued involvement with legislators, the media, and health policy formulators is a high priority for both ANA and AAOHN. AAOHN also works with related organizations such as the National Federation for Specialty Nursing Organizations to promote worker health and safety in the political arena and make nursing's presence known in governmental affairs (Haag 1991).

Government Action

The Alcohol, Drug Abuse, and Mental Health Administration of the Public Health Service (PHS) designs and promotes innovative clinical and public health strategies to treat disorders through the work site and to prevent related deficits.

- The National Institute on Alcohol Abuse and Alcoholism (NIAAA), through its employee assistance programs and Prevention Research Branch projects, addresses work site issues of alcohol abuse.
- The National Institute on Drug Abuse (NIDA), through its Office of Workplace Initiatives, provides consultation, publications, and resource referral information to employees throughout the United States.
- The National Institute of Mental Health (NIMH), through its preventive Intervention Research Center Program, develops informa-

tion about the prevention of mental disorders related to employment stress and employment transitions.

- Both the NIAAA and the NIDA are cosponsoring the inclusion of
alcohol and drug abuse information at the workplace into the curriculum for nursing education.
- The National Institute for Occupational Safety and Health
(NIOSH) provides surveillance (identification and monitoring of
disease and injury); research about work-related diseases and injuries; and dissemination of information about occupational
health hazards, potential risks, and recommendations for occupational exposures to toxic agents.

In addition, the Occupational Safety and Health Administration
(OSHA) of the Department of Labor strives to provide workers with a
healthy and safe job environment, develops safety and health standards, enforces these standards, and conducts training programs for
safety and health personnel (DHHS 1990).

Summary

A work site may be viewed as a community of employees and their families whose health and wellness extend beyond work. Work-site nurses
are community health- and wellness-oriented case managers who can
bring access to health and wellness for individuals and groups of people in ways that most health professionals cannot.

General concern and the desire for less costly and more accessible
prevention and health promotion are rising as government, private industry, and consumers explore new methods of overhauling the nation's health care delivery system. Work-site wellness programs that
teach, encourage, and help employees adopt and maintain life style
behaviors compatible with health promotion are part of the new
health care delivery system.

Appropriately, occupational and work-site nurses are no longer concerned only with first aid, work injury prevention, and levels of exposure to toxic substances. These nurses have an impact on life style behaviors that have implications for extended health and wellness for
people throughout the life span and in the community at large.

References

American Nurses Association. 1991. *Nursing's agenda for health care reform.* Kansas
City, MO: Author.
Haag, A. 1991. From the president: Governmental affairs progress continues.
AAOHN News 11(8), p. 1.

Johnson, D.R. 1991. Health promotion: The challenge to industry. In *Health at work*, eds. S.M. Weiss, J.E. Fielding, and A. Baum, pp. 29–36. Hillsdale, NJ: Lawrence Erlbaum.

Jose, W.S., II, and Anderson, D.R. 1991. Control Data's StayWell program: A health cost management strategy. In *Health at work*, eds. S.M. Weiss, J.E. Fielding, and A. Baum, pp. 49–72. Hillsdale, NJ: Lawrence Erlbaum.

U.S. Department of Health and Human Services. 1990. *Prevention '89/'90: Federal programs and progress.* Washington, DC: U.S. Government Printing Office.

U.S. Department of Health and Human Services. 1991. *Healthy people 2000: National health promotion and disease prevention objectives* (DHHS Publication No. PHS 91-50212). Washington, DC: U.S. Government Printing Office.

9

Prevention: Older Adults

Kathleen Beckman Blomquist, Ph.D., R.N., M.S.N., M.P.H.
Assistant Research Professor
Sanders-Brown Center on Aging
University of Kentucky
Lexington, Kentucky

When I was a public health nurse, an elderly client told me she would be happy as long as she had someplace to live, someone to love, and something to do. As I grow older, I realize how well she described that illusive concept, "quality of life." Americans are growing older. People over 65 years make up about 12 percent of the population and are predicted to reach 23 percent by the year 2040. Life expectancy has increased dramatically since 1900, and people who reach the age of 65 years can expect to live well into their 80s. Medical advances are extending life faster than they are slowing the onset of chronic disabling conditions.

We have added years to life, but not life to those additional years. Because disease is so prevalent in older adults (86 percent have one or more chronic diseases), preventive programs focus on maintaining health and functional independence. Although it is commonly believed that health problems in old age are inevitable, many are preventable or can be controlled (Berg and Cassells 1990). With older adults, the focus of nursing is to search for potential and nurture it to promote health and prevent disability.

Defining Successful Aging

Aging is not pathological; it is gradual and part of the developmental continuum. Who is old and the status of the elderly is culturally determined. Unfortunately, being old in America carries a stigma, in part because emphasis has been on loss and deterioration. However, research is showing that many age-associated declines (such as a carbohydrate intolerance, osteoporosis, and decline in cognitive function) can be explained by level of physical activity, diet, substance use, and an array of psychosocial factors extrinsic to the aging process. The range of heterogeneity with respect to physiological and cognitive characteristics is greater for the elderly than for any other age group, and this heterogeneity challenges program planning (Nouwen and Gaffney 1974).

Successful aging is usually defined as retaining the ability to function independently. Predictors of successful aging have been identified by several longitudinal studies. Successful aging seems to be related to rating one's health as good in middle life, having no bad outcomes for one's spouse, having good mental status, and retiring in good health. Individuals with more low-risk life style practices tend to have lower mortality rates. Moderation and balance in diet and abstinence from tobacco, alcohol, and other substances throughout life improve health in later life. Physical activity is highly related to independence in later life, and higher income is related to higher levels of functioning at older ages.

Higher education is associated with longer life, especially for women. Education and income do not seem to be associated with higher use of medical care services. Possibly, higher education affects the timing of contact. Earlier treatment and compliance with treatment promote health and prevent disability. People with more education may be more in tune with their symptoms, talk about changes with people in their support network who are also likely to be educated and knowledgeable, and find information that leads them to improve life style practices. Research needs to look at which early and middle life experiences are related to successful aging and what happens when we age as opposed to when we develop diseases (Roos and Havens 1991).

Someplace to Live

A comfortable environment is important for quality of life. Older people want to stay in their own homes as long as possible, because inability to live in one's own home is a signal that one is not able to live up to the demands of the environment and that one is handicapped either physically or mentally. Perceived control seems to contribute to successful aging, and loss of home signals loss of autonomy and control over one's own life. Elders who perceive they have the ability to make decisions regarding choice of activity, timing, and pace, report higher life satisfaction. Predictability seems to be an important factor in perception of control. The extent to which control and autonomy are encouraged or denied may be a major determinant of whether aging is successful in a number of physiologic and behavioral dimensions (Rowe and Kahn 1987).

Home Environment

Affordable housing is an issue for older people who live with reduced incomes after retirement or who may have spent their savings on medical expenses. One-third of the elderly live in poverty and women make up 72 percent of those over age 65 years who live in poverty. Social policy aimed at developing a wide range of housing options—such as in-home assistance, support for families caring for their elders, mechanisms for finding roommates to share housing and expenses, group homes, and acceptable institutions for the truly dependent—is important. Matching the characteristics of the person (assertiveness, sociability, and interpersonal and physical competence) with the characteristics of the milieu (physical layout, social climate, and opportunity for control) can be challenging.

Safe housing to prevent accidents is important. Falls resulting from unsafe physical structures; vision, hearing, and tactile losses with aging and disease processes; and side effects of medications produce devastating disability, dependence, and cost. Nurses can help elders and their families assess home environments for safety hazards and help elders make acceptable modifications that compensate for sensory losses. Medication regimens may need to be altered when side effects produce changes in equilibrium. Adequate diet at home requires safe refrigeration and cooking facilities, ability to shop, and maintenance of dental and oral health. Diet and dental care affect strength, appearance, sociability, and ability for self-care.

Community Support

A safe home is part of the environment. Elders who live in low-income areas where crime or fear of crime makes them feel vulnerable may venture out less often and become isolated. Changes in the ability to make rapid judgments in complex situations may result in motor vehicle accidents for older pedestrians and drivers. Control of crime and provision of transportation are social policy challenges to maintenance of elders' health.

Support for care givers is vital to maintaining the independence of the elderly. With increased longevity, several generations may need support simultaneously. The need for middle-age people to care for children and elders financially, logistically, and emotionally may require new networks of health and social services. Government policy also has to consider how to care for older people who cannot be maintained at home for long periods, in ways that decrease fear of impoverishment and loss of control by the elders and their families.

The Block Nurse Program in St. Paul, Minnesota, is an example of how nurses promote health by focusing on maintaining older adults in their homes (see Jamieson, Campbell, and Clark 1989). The program is a neighborhood-based system of service delivery that uses neighborhood professional and volunteer personnel to provide—directly or with other agencies—health and social services needed by residents to enable them to remain in their own homes and avoid unnecessary or premature institutionalization.

Clients are persons over 65 years of age living in the designated geographic area. Each client is assessed by a "primary block nurse," a neighborhood resident who is a public health nurse employed by the county, trained in gerontological nursing, and familiar with the community and its needs. The nurse helps the client and family determine what services are needed and develops a care plan. Home-health aide and homemaking services are provided by paid neighborhood residents called "block companions." Counseling and emotional support are offered by volunteer "befrienders" who have been trained as peer counselors.

The program uses existing resources in the community to focus on the functional, emotional, social, and educational needs of the older residents and their families. Because care is provided by three people (nurse, block companion, and befriender) who are neighborhood residents, strangers do not enter the home and informal community support networks are used. Evaluations show that the clients of the Block Nurse Program are maintained in their homes for about half the cost of nursing home care.

Someone to Love

Having someone to love implies being loved—having family and friends in a supportive network. Social support and perception of connectedness—measured by marital status, contacts with extended family and close friends, religious group membership, and other group affiliations—are related to morbidity, mortality, and perceived quality of life. Supportive care includes providing material assistance, information, sick care, and expressions of respect and love. Teaching, encouraging, and enabling are autonomy-increasing modes of support. Constraining, "doing for," and warning may convey caring, but they teach helplessness and may have negative effects on the perceived quality of life and functional abilities of older people.

Loss

Elders often outlive their friends and suffer multiple losses and loneliness in addition to anxieties related to decreased income and increased disability. The depression that results may display itself in ways unlike manifestations of depression in younger people. Depressed mood may not be apparent, but somatic symptoms that are difficult to diagnose—such as loss of appetite, energy, and ability to think and concentrate—are more common. Risk factors for depression include family or personal history of depression; changes in physical, sensory, and cognitive function; grief and bereavement over losses of family and friends; and changes in network of support including geographic isolation, unplanned retirement, and loss of loved ones and confiding relationships. Constraints on activities (such as expressions of sexuality), changes in sleep patterns, and effects of medications contribute to depression. Depression affects energy and motivation to be independent and may cause further disability.

More than half of all suicides occur in people suffering from depression, and over 20 percent of all suicides occur in persons over 65 years of age, especially white men. Suicide is preventable; most people contemplating suicide communicate their intent to at least one person and have seen their physician before the attempt. Prevention of suicide requires better recognition of persons at risk and improved mental health services for the elderly.

Important in the prevention of depression and suicide are meaningful activities designed to prevent withdrawal and social isolation. Involvement in the community is important to establishing links with other people to care about and get caring from, and who expect the older person to be there. Because most elderly people no longer work for a living and do not focus on "having" and "doing," they feel less valuable; the focus turns to "being" and "being with." The elderly often just want someone to listen to them without giving advice.

Elder Abuse

Care givers can help maintain independence for the elderly. But clashes between the desires of the elder and desires of family members can lead to neglect or violence. Over 1 million elders are abused each year, and in 86 percent of cases the abuser is a relative. Elder abuse can take the form of financial exploitation, overuse of medications (chemical restraints), threats and isolation, and physical or sexual abuse. The likely victim is a socially isolated elder who retains some independence and on whom the abuser is dependent financially. Abuse can be prevented by developing multiple ways for elders to have outside contacts, by planning financial and legal arrangements for future disability (powers of attorney, guardianship, wills, living arrangements, use of support services), and by developing community programs such as neighborhood watch, training for health professionals, and public awareness campaigns.

Community Support

The Parish Nurse Service at Second Presbyterian Church in Lexington, Kentucky is an example of the use of a social network to promote health. Many programs in churches help people stay well—e.g., regular opportunities for building friendships, experiencing help through prayer and worship, singing, studying, serving others, and being served by others. Churches promote interaction among all age groups and help decrease the age segregation found in older persons' lives. Nurses in churches provide functions historically provided by public health nurses:

- Teach and support young families as they adjust to new members.
- Offer screening programs to detect disease early and coordinate health promotion classes and support groups.
- Help elderly people and their families stay well or adjust to disabilities.
- Help families deal with physical and mental problems and crises of all sorts.
- Assist people before, during, and after hospitalization.
- Assist people in rallying health and social resources in the community.

The focus of the nurses is prevention rather than direct care.

The Parish Nurse Service is one of many services based on the foundation developed by Rev. Granger Westburg in the Lutheran churches in the Chicago area. The service is a collaborative effort of the church and the University of Kentucky College of Nursing. Ruth Berry, a member of Second Church and a faculty member at the college, spends 20 percent of her university time as parish nurse. She has devoted the majority of her efforts to developing programs that benefit older members of the church. In a series of classes held on Sunday mornings, members discussed normal aging and resources of older people with experts from the university including a geriatrician, a social worker, and a lawyer. A series of four classes for care givers resulted in monthly meetings that have an informational program but also offer important support-group activities and networking. This program is open to the community.

In addition, a Sunday morning health fair focused on heart health. A computerized health-risk appraisal with follow-up counseling was made available to members. The nurses of the church offered blood pressure screening one or two Sunday mornings each month, and they discussed nutrition, stress reduction, exercise, and medications during the screening sessions. This gave members the opportunity to request a conference with the parish nurse to talk about symptoms and accessing health care, and to ask questions about family members, so early case finding is accomplished. A recent health survey of the congregation found that interests for classes include exercise and fitness opportunities in the church, healthy eating and weight control, CPR, stress management, and humor. Several programs have been planned to address these issues.

Something to Do

Once retired, an elder is no longer "earning a living," though, culturally, "we are what we do." For some with a reasonable retirement income, success in their occupation, and ideas on how to spend their new-found time, spending time "playing" rather than working is something that has been earned. For others, feelings of uselessness interfere with healthy self-esteem.

Having something meaningful to do is important for elders. For example, a 76-year-old neighbor has a specific volunteer activity every day of the week except Saturday. She has structured her life so she has a reason to get up, get dressed, and get out of her house every day. Other people find volunteer work demeaning and without purpose. Some retirees take up golf, play the stock market, and travel—things they had dreamed of doing for years but had no time to do.

As a society, we can benefit from the expertise of elders as teachers in a variety of settings. Elders can assist in child care, nurturing both the children and their parents, and discussing and modeling parenting behaviors. Elders can work in schools, helping students learn the basics, specific skills, and how to apply these lessons to the workplace and other life activities. Elders can help middle-age people as they contemplate career changes and retirement.

Community Support

Staying in the work force is one way to maintain independence. Labor shortages are prompting employers to rethink mandatory retirement and to offer phased retirement. Many older adults are considering second and third careers and working part-time to use their skills or learn new ones. Others are pursuing cultural endeavors and educational opportunities like elderhostels and university programs. Older and younger adults benefit from taking classes together.

Retirement offers time to focus on oneself. Elders can take time to shop and prepare meals, take daily walks, or take up new physical activities such as golf or gardening. They may have more time and energy for sexual activity. If elders expect to remain active and symptom-free, when physical or cognitive problems interfere with their activities, they are likely to do something about them. If elders expect to become less mobile and feel less well, then they may not get help to prevent further disability. Learning new skills to care for oneself with a potentially disabling condition, completing the paper work involved with aging (Social Security and Medicare), and performing tasks done by one's spouse who may be disabled—all are challenges for older people.

Health Access 55+ is a nurse-managed program offered by Bartholomew County Hospital in Columbus, Indiana, and other members of the Voluntary Hospitals of America network. The program is a model for nurses working in community groups, such as senior-citizen housing centers. It is a personalized service designed to give adults 55 years old and older access to health care services and information. A nurse-coordinator answers health care and hospital questions and offers insurance claims assistance, home care assistance, and discounts for health care supplies at local merchants. Health education and screening focus on early case finding and transportation assistance, and wellness programs on topics ranging from communication and relationship building to weight control and healthy eating, along with fitness evaluation and exercise programs.

Also included are social events such as dinners and dances, concerts, and trips, giving older adults an opportunity to socialize and not be concerned about driving in unfamiliar places. Newsletters are distributed and address topics such as sexuality after age 55 years, reading prescription symbols and food labels, driving safety, promoting circulation, changes in sleep with age, and memory improvement strategies. Health Access 55+ focuses on primary prevention and health promotion as well as screening and early case finding.

Of course, health promotion activities should begin early in life to prevent development of many chronic diseases. In the past, discussion of health promotion activities has been omitted partly because it was thought that it was too late to prevent disease after age 65 years. As people live longer, there are more years to benefit from these activities. At 65 years old, men can be expected to live another 15 years and women another 19 years. Preventive efforts should be focused on modifying risky health behavior and early diagnosis matched to leading problems by age and functional status. As with younger age groups, the biggest challenge is to entice those who most need to participate—sedentary, smoking, low-income, socially isolated, sensory-impaired, or depressed individuals and those on multiple medications. Nurses search for potential in these people and nurture it.

There are some conditions for which disability is inevitable. A problem for families and communities is caring for the increasing number of older people with dementia. An example is the Helping Hand program operated by the Lexington/Bluegrass Alzheimer's Association (with support from the Robert Wood Johnson Foundation and the Alzheimer's Disease Research Center at the University of Kentucky). This day-care program for the elderly offers respite for families, intensive stimulation to maintain capacities of the elderly, resources for the families, and opportunity for the retired in the community to offer service. The five-day-per-week program is housed in a gathering room in a church and run by a small paid staff. Volunteers from the community, many of whom are elderly themselves, are trained to be "best friends" to the clients. All elderly clients, who may attend only a half-day or every day, have best friends who work with them.

Activities include chair exercises and bouncing balls or balloons around the circle, singing old favorite songs or playing mouth or percussion instruments, craft activities, storytelling, celebrating special events, and memory activities such as finding synonyms and antonyms. Children in the preschool housed in the church visit with the elders. One of the best friends who is 85 years old commented that she did not know if she was doing any good for the people in the program, but being part of the Helping Hand sure did good things for her—she learned things, felt useful, and had fun.

Prevention Benefits

Benefit-cost analyses for elderly preventive services may be more favorable than those for services for younger people, if the interventions are successful. New research has shown that older men and women benefit from smoking cessation as much as their middle-age counterparts do, adjusted for various coronary risk factors. On an aggregate basis, the older age group benefits far more, since the incidence of heart attack and death rises markedly with age. Similarly, because old people have a higher incidence of serious illnesses and death from influenza and pneumococcal pneumonia, immunization is more worthwhile for older age groups. The mortality and morbidity rates of most cancers rise sharply with age, so screening programs for older adults should generate more lives saved per 1,000 people screened. Older adults have higher risks of complications, so vigorous therapy that prevents disability may increase years of independent life. The outcome measure used for many benefit-cost determinations of health promotion programs is productive (that is, income-producing) years under 65 years of age. New measures of benefits, including disability prevention, must be considered.

Values older people place on aspects of quality of life can be determined. Educating health care professionals about the benefits of counseling older people about health promotion activities, sending persuasive media messages to them, and changing how health promotion is funded—all will promote health of the elderly. Insurance plans can include packages of preventive services based on work of the U.S. Preventive Services Task Force and other demonstrations. The focus must include long-term evaluation of the benefits of health promotion and screening activities. When screening programs are instituted, costs escalate because cases are found and treated. After several years the costs are lower because disease is discovered early and costly complications are averted or delayed (Omenn 1990).

Summary

People are living longer, but they are not necessarily living better. To accommodate the changing needs of an increasingly older society we must broaden the traditional goals of health—curing disease and preventing its occurrence—to include preventing the ill from becoming disabled and helping the disabled cope with and prevent further disability. Dealing with disease includes dealing with the consequences of disease—nursing's forte. Health professionals must believe there is quality of life for old people in order to help older individuals achieve it.

Realistically, older individuals can be expected to seek care for chronic illnesses, disabilities, and acute conditions. Development of interventions to maintain function among physically or mentally impaired older people must be a focus of health care professionals. Society should strive to empower older individuals by ensuring opportunities to participate in constructive roles and regain capabilities compromised by disease.

One cannot assume that limitations of function are the result of old age. Growing old does not necessarily mean growing frail. Nursing is the core of a system that emphasizes primary health care services—that promote and restore health—through partnerships between consumers and providers, making health care a part of community life. By ensuring them someplace to live, someone to love, and something to do, and nurturing their potential, nurses can promote high quality of life for older adults.

References

Berg, R.L., and Cassells, J.J., eds. 1990. *The second fifty years: Promoting health and preventing disability.* Washington, DC: National Academy of Sciences.

Jamieson, M., Campbell, J., and Clarke, S. 1989. Block nurse program. *The Gerontologist* 29(1), 124–127.

Nouwen, H.J.M., and Gaffney, W.J. 1974. *Aging: The fulfillment of life.* New York: Doubleday.

Omenn, G.S. 1990. Prevention and the elderly: Appropriate policies. *Health Affairs* 9(2), 80–93.

Roos, N.P., and Havens, B. 1991. Predictors of successful aging. A twelve-year study of Manitoba elderly. *American Journal of Public Health* 81(1), 63–68.

Rowe, J.W., and Kahn, F.L. 1987. Human aging: Usual and successful. *Science* 237, 143–149.

10

Research Applications in Prevention

Carolyn A. Williams, Ph.D., R.N., F.A.A.N.
Dean and Professor
College of Nursing
University of Kentucky
Lexington, Kentucky

Within the past 20 years, concern for fitness in America for the year 2000 and beyond has mobilized a number of groups to focus attention on prevention. Of particular importance has been a series of federal initiatives that have resulted in the contemporary effort to establish national goals for health promotion and disease prevention, *Healthy People 2000* (DHHS 1991).

In this chapter, three broad topics are discussed. First, the magnitude and nature of preventable mortality are presented and terminology used in discussing prevention will be summarized. The second part of the chapter focuses on the application of current knowledge about prevention in community settings. The chapter concludes with comments about future directions in practice and research to guide preventive strategies, with particular attention to priority topics for nurse researchers.

How important are preventive strategies? What if someone told you that it was highly possible that 63 percent of the deaths which occur in a given year were premature? Can such a thing be so? If it is true, why isn't more being done about it? Amler and Dull (1987) documented a health policy effort of the Carter Center of Emory University which had as its objective "to highlight missed opportunities for preventing premature deaths and unnecessary disability in the United States using prevention strategies already in hand" (p. vii). An expert panel selected health problems that represented significant mortality and morbidity and that were amenable to reduction. The specific criteria used in the selection were: "1) point prevalence and secular trends, 2) severity of health impact and cost, 3) severity of intervention using current scientific or operational knowledge, 4) feasibility of such intervention, and, 5) generic applicability of such intervention to other health problems" (p. 182).

The health problems selected for study were alcohol dependency and abuse, arthritis and musculoskeletal diseases, cancer, cardiovascular diseases, dental diseases, depression, diabetes mellitus, digestive diseases, unintended pregnancy and infant mortality and morbidity, unintentional injury, and violence (homicide, domestic violence, and suicide). Analysis showed that these broad health problems accounted for 94.4 percent of the total deaths in the United States in 1980 and 78 percent of the potential life lost before the age of 65 years. Clearly, the stunning information is that 63 percent of the deaths that occurred in 1980 were attributed to identified precursors deemed amenable to change, or to put it another way, were thought to be preventable given present knowledge.

It was estimated that three precursors, tobacco use, high blood pressure, and obesity together accounted for 73 percent of preventable deaths. Based on 1980 data, it was also estimated that 75 percent of the years of life lost before the age of 65 years can be attributed to four precursors: injury risks, alcohol/tobacco use, and gaps in primary prevention. The study concluded that "the burden of premature death in the United States in the 1980s is large and, in large measure, preventable. . . . Whether measured by crude deaths or by years of life lost before the age of 65, approximately two-thirds of deaths in the United States are attributable to a preventable precursor and thus are potentially unnecessary, or premature" (p. 187).

The central challenge of *Healthy People 2000* is "to implement what is already known about promoting health and preventing disease" (DHHS 1991, p. 6). Thus, the objectives that have been set and the strategies projected for attaining them are based on previous research conducted by investigators representing a broad range of disciplines.

The objectives are organized into three broad categories according to the type of preventive interventions involved: health promotion, health protection, and prevention services. *Health promotion* activities involve community and individual measures fostering life styles that maintain and enhance well-being and health. Personal choices related to physical activity and fitness, nutrition, tobacco/alcohol use, family planning, mental health, and violent and abusive behavior can be influenced by health promotion strategies.

Health protection refers to strategies designed to protect defined population groups. Such measures foster changes in the physical and social environment that are designed to improve health and well-being. Such changes are frequently brought about through legislation and government regulation. Examples include strategies designed to ensure the safety of food and drugs and promote safety in occupational environments and in the broader environment. *Preventive health services* are directed at individuals to prevent the development of specific disorders or diseases. They are usually implemented in clinical settings.

The terms "primary," "secondary," and "tertiary" prevention are frequently used in discussions on prevention. The question of how these terms relate to health promotion, health protection, and preventive health services may arise. *Primary prevention* is targeted on intervention before negative changes occur. General health promotion (for example, exercise and good nutrition) and specific protection from defined health problems (for example, immunizations) are considered primary preventive measures. *Secondary prevention* is aimed at detecting problems early and intervening quickly, and *tertiary prevention* focuses on limitation of disability and rehabilitation (for example, speech therapy for stroke patients).

Application of Knowledge in Community Settings

Regardless of one's area of specialization or the setting in which an individual practices, there are numerous opportunities to engage in preventive activities. However, for those practicing in a community setting, prevention should be a major item on the practice agenda. A considerable database already exists to provide direction for the provision of preventive services. Because it is necessary to be selective in this discussion, only a few examples can be provided. Because of its uniqueness, the work of the U.S. Preventive Services Task Force is highlighted.

The task force, an interdisciplinary group, worked for several years to produce a set of guidelines for providing preventive services in clinical settings, particularly community-based clinical settings such as neighborhood health centers, primary care centers, health departments, clinics, and offices of providers such as nurse practitioners and physicians. The unique feature of the task force's work is the strategy used to evaluate the research literature to identify those preventive measures that can be substantiated on the basis of research. This process, detailed in the task force's major publication, *Guide to Clinical Preventive Services* (U.S. Preventive Services Task Force 1989), resulted in recommendations based on a careful review of the research literature and provided information regarding the quality of the underlying database.

The task force's recommendations can be grouped into those that relate to counseling (primary prevention), immunizations, and drug prophylactics (primary prevention for groups defined by age or other risk factors), and screening activities and focused examinations (secondary prevention). For each of the conditions for which preventive recommendations were developed, a detailed discussion is presented that includes statements on the burden of suffering for the problem to be prevented, efficacy of the proposed intervention, and, if available, the recommendations of other groups. In addition, a series of charts is provided, listing specific services that should be considered for patients in different age groups during a periodic health examination. In selecting items for these charts, two factors were considered: the leading causes for mortality and morbidity in the age group, and the potential effectiveness of the clinical intervention in affecting outcomes.

Much of the attention of health professionals who work in community health settings is focused on those patients who actually appear in the clinical environment. However, there have been a number of clinical trials or demonstration projects that have assessed the effectiveness of community-based strategies for reducing the risk of health problems in people not defined as patients.

Most pronounced among these are projects focused on the prevention of cardiovascular diseases. These large, epidemiology-oriented studies can be grouped into two major categories. The more traditional focuses on sub-populations, such as men of a certain age group. They involve a screening process, and for those found to have high levels of specified risk factors (for example, blood lipids or high blood pressure), interventions are provided to change risk profiles. Such studies use the "high-risk" approach, which means they are directed to individuals in the higher range of the distribution of one or more risk factors. Studies such as the Multiple Risk Factor Intervention Trial (MRFIT) (MRFIT Research Group 1982) fall into this group and have shown the benefits of reducing risk factors in the prevention of cardiovascular mortality and morbidity.

Of growing interest is a second group of studies that focus on the entire population—the free-living population—and involve activities that affect the total social environment at the community level. The Stanford Five-City Project is one such study in which mass communication strategies for health education—involving television, radio, newspapers, and other media—were used in an effort to reach all segments of the community. Also, face-to-face education strategies, dealing with the need for exercise and the need to reduce and eliminate tobacco use and decrease dietary fat, were directed at all members of the community, regardless of their risk profiles (Farquhar et al. 1990).

The total-population approach is gaining attention because of what are now viewed as more positive outcomes than those achieved by the high-risk approach. Although there is a clustering of deaths in those with high levels of cardiovascular risk factors, the majority of deaths in a population that can be attributed to cardiovascular diseases are among those who have average or moderately elevated risk levels. Thus, the population approach focused on changing the distribution of risk factors for an entire population in a more positive direction affects more people who are affected by the problem, resulting in a better outcome at the population level (Kottke, Puska, Salonen, Tuomilehto, and Nissinen 1985).

Key differences between the high-risk and the population approaches include the prominent role of mass communication messages in the population approach and the way that screening activities are handled. In the high-risk approach, the purpose of screening is to find people with high-risk factors and to initiate early intervention such as intensive education or pharmacological treatment. In contrast, in the population approach, the goal is to identify where the individual is with regard to risk factors and to educate the client in ways that will facilitate a change in behavior. These two approaches are not mutually exclusive and, in fact, in community-wide studies, the high-risk approach has been subsumed as one of the strategies used. The key point is that community-wide strategies are not limited to focusing on high-risk individuals.

Future Directions

Practice

A major focus for future activity should be on finding ways to act on the knowledge base presently available, as well as encouraging research activity to inform prevention decision-making. As has been presented, there is considerable information at hand that, if used in practice, could favorably influence the health status of the population. Thus, positive action at the level of individual clinicians and those responsible for programs is needed. Professionals in clinical settings and those managing community-focused efforts need to review the way business is being done and move toward implementing preventive strategies shown to be effective. For example, there is much to be gained from incorporating information in the report of the Preventive Services Task Force into clinical services offered by primary care providers. Although cost issues are frequently offered as reasons for not implementing certain strategies, health professionals need to break down such barriers and work toward finding ways to provide such services at affordable rates.

Another important goal for the future is to focus more attention on health promotion and protection activities that involve community-wide strategies and strategies that target population groups such as those at work sites and in schools. Currently, health professionals, even those employed in public health agencies, are directing vast resources and energy into the provision of clinical services, only a part of which are preventive. For prevention to have a major impact on the population, more energy must be directed to community-wide strategies and programs that have impact on populations where they are.

Community-wide initiatives—such as the Healthy Cities Project of Indiana (Kellogg Foundation 1988) and other efforts oriented to mobilizing community resources and developing partnerships between constituencies in the community and health professionals—are needed to implement preventive strategies that will have an impact on the population. Another need is to work toward developing public policies at all levels of government to promote healthy environments and healthy behaviors.

To summarize, three important goals for practitioners and public health specialists are:

- to incorporate more preventive strategies into the provision of services in community-based clinical settings.
- to direct more attention to community-wide preventive strategies for developing healthy environments and healthy behaviors.
- to be involved actively in the development of public policies that support healthy environments and healthy behaviors.

Research

There is a discouraging discrepancy between the primary role that nurses frequently play in the provision of preventive services to population groups in the community and in clinical settings, and research to guide the nature of the interventions. This is particularly apparent in areas such as prenatal care, strategies designed to prevent unintentional pregnancies in adolescents, and teaching and counseling to encourage smoking cessation, healthy nutrition, and positive exercise behaviors. For example, a review of the literature related to the prevention of unintended adolescent pregnancies (Fielding and Williams 1990) indicated that in a number of the programs and demonstration projects designed to prevent unintended adolescent pregnancies, nurses actually provided much of the care. Yet very few nurses were involved in the research aspects of the projects, and there was very little information regarding specific strategies found effective.

Thus, on one hand there is a problem of epidemic proportions, a problem to which much professional time is given in a variety of programs, and yet the research base for such programs is quite limited. The research to date indicates some success with both community- and school-based services that improve the access of adolescents to educational and contraceptive services (Fielding and Williams 1990).

When one considers the community-wide studies on cardiovascular disease mentioned earlier, it is clear that providers such as nurses are active participants in providing much of the ongoing screening and educational activities in these efforts. Yet nurse researchers have not been involved, and nurse researchers have not given much attention to research directed to community-wide populations. Although there are a number of reasons for this state of affairs, the following future research directions might be particularly beneficial to improving the knowledge base for prevention.

- Attention should focus on high-prevalence problem areas in which nurses are already involved in dealing with the target populations (for example, with adolescents, to prevent unintentional pregnancies, with school children to develop healthy attitudes and behaviors related to sexual activity).
- Studies should advance knowledge in the design of community-wide strategies for health promotion and health protection. These studies would be helpful in guiding program developers in evolving partnerships with community groups to effect positive behavioral changes as well as to improve public health policy.

References

Amler, R.W., and Dull, H.B., eds. 1987. *Closing the gap: The burden of unnecessary illness.* New York: Oxford University Press.

Farquhar, J.W., Fortmann, S.P., Flora, J.A., Taylor, B., Haskell, W.L., Williams, P.T., Maccoby, N., and Wood, P.D. 1990. Effects of community-wide education on cardiovascular disease risk factors: The Stanford five-city project. *Journal of the American Medical Association* 264(3), 359–365.

Fielding, J.E., and Williams, C.A. 1990. Unwanted teenage pregnancy: A U.S. perspective. In *Preventing disease: Beyond the rhetoric,* eds. Goldbloom, R.P.B. and Lawrence, R.S., pp. 94–100. New York: Springer-Verlag.

Kellogg Foundation funds three-year "Healthy Cities Indiana" project. 1988 (December). *American Journal of Public Health* 78(12), p. 5.

Kottke, T.E., Puska, P., Salonen, J.T., Tuomilehto, J., and Nissinen, A. 1985. *American Journal of Epidemiology* 121(5), 697–704.

Multiple Risk Factor Intervention Trial Research Group. 1982. Multiple risk factor intervention trial: Risk factor changes and mortality results. *Journal of the American Medical Association* 248(12), 1465–1477.

U.S. Department of Health and Human Services. 1991. *Healthy people 2000: National health promotion and disease prevention objectives.* Washington, DC: U.S. Government Printing Office.

U.S. Preventive Services Task Force. 1989. *Guide to clinical preventive services: An assessment of the effectiveness of 169 interventions.* Baltimore: Williams & Wilkins.

11

Health Promotion: Public Policy Goal

Gloria R. Smith, Ph.D., R.N., F.A.A.N.
Program Director and Coordinator
Health Programs
Kellogg Foundation
Battle Creek, Michigan

and

Ruby L. Wesley, Ph.D., R.N.
Director of Nursing Practice
The Rehabilitation Institute of Michigan
Assistant Professor
College of Nursing
Wayne State University
Detroit, Michigan

The Clinton Administration has pushed health care reform to the top of the nation's domestic policy agenda. The heightened debate on the issue of a national health plan is fueled by the belief that only a national framework holds the promise of universal access to affordable basic health services. Universal access to affordable basic health services cannot by itself, however, make us a healthy nation. The current debate fails to focus on the contribution of disease prevention and health promotion to the affordability of universal access. Much less is it driven by a common vision of a healthy people.

Medical care is necessary but not sufficient for the attainment of health. Limiting the concept of "access" to "access to medical care" will have two negative effects. It will deny the medical care system potential savings from prevention and it will rob resources from other sectors whose contributions are also necessary for the attainment of health. If we as a people want to attain universal access we must recast the policy question and ask, "Access to what?" The focus should shift from access to curative care alone to access to a reformed health system encompassing prevention, protection, and promotion.

The current debate emphasizes organizing, financing, and paying for medical care. Familiar topics today are voluntary versus mandatory participation in health care purchasers' alliances, single-payer versus multiple-payer models, and reliance on managed care, global budgeting, and workplace coverage. Clinical preventive services are on the sidelines, while health protection and promotion are virtually invisible.

The terms of the visible debate that has taken shape obscure the fact that the Clinton Plan actually holds out some promise for directing appropriate resources toward promoting healthy individuals and communities. On paper, the Clinton Plan offers opportunity for progress toward national objectives for the health of the U.S. population. Without a change in the terms of the debate, this promise will likely prove illusory.

This debate is taking place because hard facts could no longer be ignored. From 1980 to 1989, the percentage of the U.S. gross national product (GNP) consumed by health care expenditures rose from 5.3 percent to 11.6 percent (Levit, Lazenby, Letsch, and Cowan 1991). In spite of this impressive outlay of resources, universal access to basic health care services remains an intractable problem. More than 35 million Americans are uninsured and 19 million are under-insured. More than one-third of the uninsured are children. There is no comprehensive insurance coverage to pay for long-term care expenses, a growing problem. The future for retiree health plans looks dismal. Young, old, working, nonworking—there are barriers to care for too many Americans.

The links between costs of care and access to care seem obvious, so there has been great preoccupation with containing and reducing costs. The cost-containment imperative has led to massive restructuring in the delivery of physician and hospital services. This response, however, has not been viewed as adequate as national spending for health has exceeded the rate of growth of the GNP. Anticipated savings have not been squeezed from system changes to give relief to employers, customers, or taxpayers, or to pass along to subsidize access for those needing assistance.

In this environment, a national framework has come to be seen as the only realistic option for attaining universal access to care at an affordable cost. Clearly, change is imminent, more than ever before. It does not seem likely that Americans will become "place-bound"; i.e., held in place by company health insurance plans. The prospect of "job lock" may be very frightening to workers of all ages. The interests of insured and under-insured workers, the individually insured, and the uninsured are coming together in the health policy arena.

The United States spent $604.1 billion on health care in 1989 (Levit et al. 1991). It is estimated that 3 percent of all health care expenditures is spent on preventive services. The major policy document providing direction during the 1980s was *Promoting Health/Preventing Disease: Objectives for the Nation* (U.S. Department of Health, Education and Welfare 1980). The document outlined objectives for 1990 and contained 15 priority areas for program development at the local, state, and federal levels:

- accident prevention and injury control, control of stress and violent behavior
- family planning
- fluoridation and dental health
- high blood pressure
- immunization
- misuse of alcohol and drugs
- nutrition
- occupational safety and health
- physical fitness and exercise
- pregnancy and infant health
- sexually transmitted diseases
- smoking and health
- surveillance and control of infectious disease, and,
- toxic agent control.

A survey conducted by the Michigan Department of Public Health (1988) indicated that $1.6 billion had been targeted by the states to meet the 1990 objectives in the 15 program areas. Although this was a significant expenditure within the context of state and territorial health agency budgets, it was a minuscule outlay for primary prevention within the context of health care expenditures exceeding a half trillion dollars or more.

Healthy People 2000 (DHHS 1990), the document that follows the 1990 objectives for the nation, contains an expanded list of 21 priority areas in three broad categories: 1) health promotion strategies related to individual life style; 2) health protection strategies related to environmental or regulatory measures for the protection of large population groups; and 3) preventive services strategies related to counseling, screening, and interventions for selected disease conditions and services. The twenty-second priority is to establish a surveillance and data management system for the accomplishment of the health objectives.

A trend among policy makers has been to demand that individuals assume responsibility for personal and family health. Unfortunately, that focus is too narrow, aimed only at reducing access to or demand for insurance benefits. As policy makers move closer to finally taking action, more attention needs to be focused on a health care system with the capacity to help people remain healthy.

Milio (1983) emphasized that too often primary prevention is confused with primary health care. Primary prevention is the prevention of disease, disability, or ill health, whereas primary health care is the general first contact with the health care system. If people are to live healthier lives, use health care services appropriately and judiciously, and contribute to the formation and maintenance of caring communities, policies must be enacted to give them the necessary incentives, knowledge, and tools. The current policy debate for a national health plan focuses on reforms that will not accomplish this.

Harrington (1990) categorized proposals for a national health plan into three groups:

1. Incremental expansion of the existing public programs (Medicare and Medicaid).
2. Mandatory requirements for employers to offer private health insurance to employees.
3. A comprehensive national health plan similar to the one in Canada.

To this we must add the Clinton national health plan, which is comprehensive, contains mandates and, unlike the Canadian model, is multiple-payer, not single-payer. In addition to the Chafee alternative to the Clinton Plan, another voluntary approach being advanced is the medical IRA.

A comprehensive national health plan offers the greatest potential for health-promoting approaches with strong support for primary prevention. Such health-promoting approaches are in the Clinton Plan, but whether they will survive the policy making process in a meaningful way is an open question. The plan offers a ray of hope because of its Public Health Initiative, Prevention Research Initiative, data-system linkages to serve both medical care and public health, provisions for school-based health services, and loans to foster development of community-based health plans. The plan's inclusion of health education and clinical preventive services in the benefit package is encouraging. The need to train or retrain health professionals with true community-health orientations is recognized in the plan.

The great uncertainty is whether these public health initiatives have the opportunity to be funded and whether priorities will be set that channel appropriate resources to them. The debate preceding introduction of the Clinton Plan is illuminating. A brief discussion of two of the most recent proposals portending a narrow thrust in the area of primary prevention follows.

In June 1991, the Blue Cross/Blue Shield Association (BCBSA), which represents a major segment of the health insurance industry, released a statement to the press on new recommended clinical guidelines for adult services. The guidelines were the result of three years of collaboration between the American College of Physicians (ACP) and the BCBSA (1991). A survey of Blue Cross/Blue Shield (BCBS) plans showed that 70 percent either have marketed or are developing screening and health education programs for targeted areas, e.g., pregnancy, newborn, and well-child. Only 4 percent of BCBS plans reported that disease prevention and health promotion are among employers' top three priorities, even though costs for such services are modest. Monthly costs for adult preventive and screening services are estimated to be approximately $3 for an individual and $7.50 for a family.

The Institute of Medicine (1988) published a report on the future of public health. Responding to the mandate to examine the state of public health and policy pertaining to the health of the public, problems were categorized into three areas: immediate crises, such as AIDS and health care for the indigent; injuries, teen pregnancy, high blood pressure, smoking and substance abuse; and looming problems, such as hazardous waste and Alzheimer's disease. The study concluded that poor intergovernmental relationships result in a lack of leadership at many levels, a blurred vision of the mission of public health, and limited finances for public health care. New, enlightened, and powerful directions for public health policy were not forthcoming.

Health Policy Conceptual Model

Nursing's Agenda for Health Care Reform (ANA 1991) has been developed and endorsed by more than 65 professional nursing organizations. The nursing community has called for a basic core of essential health care services to be made available. The focus is a call for a shift in resources from illness and cure to more appropriate allocations aimed at wellness and care. The basic components of this agenda include a restructured health care system focusing on access, consumer responsibility, and cost-effective therapeutic options. The organizations also want a federally defined standard package of essential health care services provided and financed through public and private plans. Another key element of this proposal is a call for planned change to anticipate health service needs that coincide with changing national demographics. This agenda for health care reform is another positive step toward support and establishment of national health care policies to ensure the nation's health.

Based on documented evidence of past successful campaigns to eliminate or reduce health risks, some policy researchers have recommended a different approach to health policy and new health promotion models.

De Leeuw (1989) proposed a model that places the variable of health promotion within a societal context (Figure 11.1). This model can be useful in examining health prevention and health policy development. The underlying assumptions of this model are that:

- The health sector has generally been isolated from other societal and policy sectors.
- The promotion of people's health has thus far, from government perspectives, been a matter of personal life style modification.
- The actual causes of health are intricate, intertwined, varied, and interdependent—in short, complex.
- Social policy is the largest determinant of health.

The issue, therefore, is not just health care organization policy, but overall policies with health consequences.

The model has five sections within its parameters. On the side is the problem definer field, the area where the problem is formulated and preferred options and interventions are filtered through the area of intermediate determinants (these two areas make up the "policy making environment"). The intermediate determinants include cultural, social, economic, organizational, and societal constraints and stimuli. The health interventions or programs decided on are influenced by the determinants, which are the services that need to be provided, the individual and collective behavior, and support systems formulated in the policy making environment. Depending on the distribution or equity of the interventions and programs, a favorable health situation will be present in a given population.

There are two examples that demonstrate social policies with healthy consequences. One is the health care issue of primary dental problems and the other is the hazards of smoking. The model can be used to examine policy making on these issues. Tooth decay was identified as a major health problem affecting 90 percent of Americans. Early research indicated that fluoridated water would prevent almost two-thirds of the dental caries. With this evidence available, it was determined that 17.6 million days of disability a year, or close to one day per ten people, could be avoided (Milio 1983).

A variety of interventions were proposed to affect this problem, including pressure groups advocating change, health education programs in schools, and institution of policies related to fluoridated water supplied in communities. Because the distribution of this intervention could address the needs of only 40 percent of Americans, additional resources were allocated. Development of toothpaste with fluoride, mouthwashes that reduce plaque buildup, and a massive advertising campaign took place to reach the rest of America.

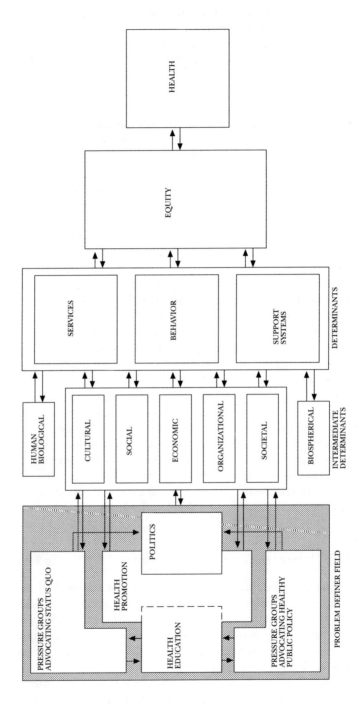

Fig. 11.1. A Model to Position Health Promotion in the Societal Context.

It is clear from this example that the proposed programs and interventions that were addressed in the policy making area ultimately were affected by the service made available, consumer behavior, and the support systems put in place. Equitable distribution of the program and interventions resulted in effective primary dental health care and avoidance of approximately 85 days of disability per 1,000 individuals.

Another example of the usefulness of the model in examining health in a societal context is the reduction of cigarette smoking or changing smoking behavior to reduce the risk of chronic disease. The U.S. Surgeon General stated that adults smoked an average of 3,900 cigarettes during 1979 and that 32 percent of American adults were smokers. After the risks were identified—cardiovascular disease, cancer, stroke, hypertension, and emphysema—a variety of interventions and programs were proposed and implemented (Milio 1983). Using the model, and progressing from the problem definer field to the intermediate determinants, we see tremendous pressure for positive change from consumers.

However, the powerful tobacco industry lobbyists opposed many of the proposed interventions. Filter-tip cigarettes were promoted as being safer and brands lower in tar and nicotine flourished in the marketplace. Various social policies affected the reduction of cigarette smoking as well, including no smoking at many work sites, no smoking on airplane flights of less than two hours, no advertising of cigarettes on television, massive health education programs on the hazards of smoking, stop-smoking clinics, surgeon general's warnings on the product itself, increased cost of and taxes on cigarettes, and penalties on many health or life insurance policies for smoking.

Clearly, the constraints on cigarette consumption (33 percent drop) were operationalized in the intermediate determinants and determinants areas of the model. These policies, interventions, and programs have resulted in reduction in the number of cigarette smokers (21 percent drop) and improved health for the nation.

Health Protection or Health Promotion: Public Policy Goal

The goal of a healthy nation has not been realized in the 1990s, but strategies for change have demonstrated a measure of success for promotion of a healthy community. But strategies that focus only on screening or on providing basic health care services or reducing risk factors for individuals are not enough to bring about desired change in the nation's health status.

What are needed are appropriate resources directed toward promoting healthy individuals and communities. This can be accomplished only through a combination of strategies that include incentives for individuals to assume greater responsibility for maintaining and protecting their own health and the health of their families, universal access to health services, and population- or community-based interventions directed toward improving the health status of the community. The goal for improved health status for Americans, commensurate with the wealth, technology, expertise, and experience of our institutions, is attainable.

While, with the Clinton Plan, national policy thinking is progressing toward recognition that "social policy is the largest determinant of health," the final outcome of the debate may narrowly focus on benefits, eligibility, financing, cost-control, and administration. The resources necessary for universal access and the massive structural transformation proposed to bring it about may overshadow—and consume available dollars and energy for—significant redirection and strengthening in public health, prevention, and protection. The process and the cost will likely push promotion and protection to the periphery.

Many may not notice, but the ultimate cost of marginalizing what should be central may be high. The forces and factors in public health, prevention, and community development thus diminished might prove to be "but for" forces and factors—but for their absence, the affordability of universal access might have been achieved through taking the lowest-cost route to individual and community health.

References

American College of Physicians and Blue Cross and Blue Shield Association. 1991. *Clinical recommendations on adult screening services.* Chicago, IL: Authors.

American Nurses Association. 1991. *Nursing's agenda for health care reform.* Kansas City, MO: Author.

De Leeuw, E. 1989. *The sane revolution health promotion: Backgrounds, scope, prospects.* The Netherlands: Van Gorcum, Assen/Maastricht.

Harrington, C. 1990. Policy options for a national health care plan. *Nursing Outlook* 38(5), 223–228.

Institute of Medicine. 1988. *The future of public health.* Washington, DC: National Academy Press.

Levit, K.R., Lazenby, H.C., Letsch, S.W., and Cowan, C.A. 1991. National health care spending, 1989. *Health Affairs* 10(1), 117–130.

Milio, N. 1983. *Primary care and the public's health: Judging impacts, goals, and policies.* Lexington, MA: D.C. Heath and Co.

Michigan Department of Public Health. 1988. *Pursuing the 1990 objectives for promoting health/preventing disease: An assessment of state and territorial health agency initiatives.* Lansing, MI: Author.

U.S. Department of Health, Education and Welfare. 1980. *Promoting health/preventing disease: Objectives for the nation.* Washington, DC: U.S. Government Printing Office.

U.S. Department of Health and Human Services Public Health Service. 1990. *Healthy people 2000: National health promotion and disease prevention objectives.* Washington, DC: U.S. Government Printing Office.

12

Prevention Made Visible for the Future

Ruth N. Knollmueller, Ph.D., R.N.
Former Assistant Director
Visiting Nurse and Home Care, Inc.
Waterbury, Connecticut

—An editor friend of mine, now in her 70s, tells how she has spent most of her life eating the wrong food, smoking too much, drinking some, and leading a sedentary life style. The one thing she did do annually was see an ophthalmologist for an eye examination because her work depended on her maintaining good vision. The irony is that she now suffers from a degenerative eye disorder while her life style seems to have had little effect on her current health.

—The newspaper headline reads, "Tetanus Victim Saved in Hospital Emergency Room . . . Doctors and Nurses Heroes." Where is the applause for community health nurses and physicians from the thousands of "saved" people who have received immunization for tetanus and other communicable diseases?

—The media lists the salaries of physicians and surgeons who correct essentially preventable conditions (cardiovascular problems, neoplasms in the lung, repair of traumatic injuries, and so on), with nary a mention of what the public health physician earns.

—The cohort of nurses working in community health nursing and public health settings, as well as nurses enrolled in graduate programs of the same major specialty, is small compared to that of nurses working in institutional settings or attending graduate programs in other specialties.

Discouraging? Clinical practice outcomes for prevention and health promotion are often more noticeable because of their absence. The seeming invisibility and "softness" of prevention actions in health care delivery define a central problem when funding and other support is sought to provide these services. Evidence is prolific that prevention is necessary and that it should be a top priority of most health care service providers. Consider, for instance, the Institute of Medicine (1988) report that stated, "History teaches us that an organized community effort to prevent disease and promote health is both valuable and effective" (p. 17).

Further, there are numerous national and international publications, to which most public health providers and politicians subscribe, that have repeatedly emphasized prevention and health promotion as an essential ingredient of health care—e.g., *Global Strategy for Health for All by the Year 2000* (World Health Organization 1977); *Healthy People, the Surgeon General's Report on Health Promotion and Disease Prevention* (DHHS 1979); *Healthy People 2000, National Health Promotion and Disease Prevention Objectives* (Office of Assistant Secretary for Health and Surgeon General 1990); and *Healthy Communities 2000 Model Standards* (American Public Health Association [APHA] 1991). These documents are stellar in their focus on prevention and health promotion for the populations identified. We certainly are not at a loss for a professional road map and for official publications to push for prevention and health promotion as legitimate health service goals.

Politics of Prevention and Health Promotion

There is continuing rhetoric concerning the disarray in our current health care system. Proposed remedies for Congress to consider are numerous each year and growing, anxious special interest groups spend large sums of money to preserve the territory of the known and control the profit in health care delivery.

Virtually all proposals for changing the health care system focus on how to pay for the services rather than articulating the scope of the services to be provided. Needless to say, the costing methodology must be determined. But for taxpayers to support the program eventually developed by Congress, they must know what they are buying. Is it more of the same, i.e., coverage for only acute conditions and for the selected technology that is deemed appropriate for reimbursement with minimal, if any, prevention and health promotion services covered?

There are such persuasive data that prevention is *the* primary cost-effective approach to health care that one wonders what the problem is. A lead article in *Time* Magazine (1991) stated that, "the health-care system devotes so much of its resources to last-minute miracles that it neglects the more mundane realm of preventative medicine, where many terrible illnesses could be halted sooner or avoided altogether."

Mundane? By whose account? Certainly not to a community health nurse who has saved countless lives and avoided untold misery and cost through the provision of immunization for diphtheria, pertussis, tetanus, polio, measles, mumps, and the like; or who has informed the pregnant woman of a way to care for herself during eclampsia; or who has advised the male worker of an intervention to care for his hypertension, thus avoiding costly medical care and potential disability.

By way of example, the savings achieved by preventing a hip fracture in an adult for the first year of treatment and rehabilitation is estimated to be $40,000. Prevention of cervical cancer treatment could save $28,000 in the first year, and preventing lung cancer treatment may save $29,000 in the first year (DHHS, p. 5). Unfortunately, our usual perspective on the issue of the economics of prevention and health promotion is captured in what it costs rather than in what is saved.

Typically, and not surprisingly, nurses have been the leading health professionals in providing prevention and health promotion services for individuals, families, and communities. It has been the legacy of community health nurses to be involved directly in prevention and health promotion activities, integrating this content into clinical practice, often without allocated funding. This reputation has made it easy for officials to take for granted that nurses will do the necessary work to meet prevention objectives with our assurances of adequate funding, materials, and recognition.

In the fall of 1990, HHS formally released *Healthy People 2000.* The nearly 300 objectives in 22 priority areas are both comprehensive and appropriate, and identify populations at risk for disease, disability, or premature death. Clearly, *Healthy People 2000* and *Healthy Communities 2000* are important political and practical tools to implement prevention and health promotion goals. These documents outline specific objectives to implement care. For example, "Reduce the maternal mortality rate to no more than 3.3 per 100,000 live births from a baseline in 1987 of 6.6 per 100,000" (DHHS 1990, p. 37) is a reasonable and appropriate goal.

An example of a *Healthy Communities 2000* objective for care in the home is specified by the local agency selecting a target year when "the community will be served by a program to increase awareness of the availability, scope, and sources of home care services and their appropriate use" (APHA 1991, p. 238). Along with this objective are indicators to evaluate how this is accomplished. The indicators for this objective are: the existence of information and a referral program in the community; referrals from acute, long-term care, and mental health facilities to home health agencies; and referrals to the home care agency from non-institutional sources such as family, self, other community agencies, and health care providers. The focus is on prevention and health promotion using the available community and public health agencies to achieve the desired outcomes.

The three broad public health goals for *Healthy People 2000* are to increase the span of healthy life for Americans, reduce health disparities among Americans, and achieve access to preventive services for all Americans.

The broad public health goals for *Healthy Communities 2000* are to emphasize health outcomes, and to have flexibility to allow communities to establish objectives and to develop strategies pertinent to their situations.

The absence of funding methodology is deliberate, leaving it up to those of us in the industry to lobby and develop funding mechanisms for these services. With good data and solid approaches for implementing these services, we must accept the funding challenge.

Possibilities for Prevention and Health Promotion Services

When considering future possibilities for our practice in public health, I find myself pushing traditional boundaries outward, delving into some of my own inventions. Is it really such an unlikely scenario to imagine health insurance companies requiring each subscriber to participate actively in programs of prevention and health promotion to be eligible for certain coverage? Such a requirement would mean a critical role for the community health nurse, with a creative and solid approach to the practice of prevention, developing programs with measurable outcome objectives, perhaps using the two most current tools, *Healthy People 2000* and *Healthy Communities 2000* as the curriculum guides. Certainly the insurance industry will want only credible prevention content, and a system may need to be developed that is similar to the current one for approving professional continuing education.

There are many methods for presenting this content, in addition to conventional ones. One typical example would be a subscriber attending workshops and conferences on topics pertinent to his or her health needs, placing the subscriber into a "safer" risk pool by providing information helpful in making positive life style changes. Other approaches can include the media; perhaps a prevention and health promotion television channel sponsored by the government or a private group, through which appropriate information will be made available and to which a person could tune in for either watching or interactive viewing. The possibilities are endless if prevention and health promotion are supported officially and, yes, commercially. Such an endeavor cannot be undertaken by the public sector alone. Will public health and community health nursing be leaders in this?

We now have around-the-clock channels on television for news, sports, weather, and cartoons. Why not an around-the-clock public prevention and health promotion television station? There may be accountability of both the provider of the information and the active response from the participant should there be a tie-in with health insurance coverage. The prevention information should be presented in languages appropriate for the geographic area receiving the radio or television program. In some areas that would include but not be limited to programming in Spanish, French, Native American languages, and sign language for the visual media and telecommunication devices for the deaf (TDD). The content could be targeted to those with minimal reading and comprehension skills as well as those with more formal education.

What if you were invited to give the name of a community health nurse for consideration for the cover story article of *Time* Magazine's person of the year? Or you are asked by a member of your congressional delegation to suggest a community health nurse who could address a congressional committee or specialized United Nations body concerning preventive health care concerns? How prepared are we to respond?

One would expect that, in the future, funding for services and materials will be forthcoming because prevention and health promotion are so effective. It makes sense politically, economically, and professionally. But it is a medical emergency that gets the headlines, not the mundane but essential preventive work that nurses do to avoid most communicable diseases and other disorders. Rarely, if ever, does the public media credit nurses with directly saving lives or preventing disease. For instance, the patient who arrives in the hospital emergency room with a diagnosis of polio is "saved" by medical intervention. There is no idea that thousands of people have been prevented from contracting this disease because nurses provided the proper intervention through immunization.

Wouldn't it be splendid to read headlines in major newspapers that said, "United States Owes Healthier Life Styles to Community Health Nurses," or "Home Health Care Turns to Prevention by Nurses as First Line of Health Defense," or "Medicaid and Medicare Pay Nurses for Health Promotion Services," or "Public Health and Community Health Nurses Save Lives."

Prevention and Methods of Health Care Delivery

Popular labels these days for some forms of health care delivery are "case management," "managed care," and "managed competition"; these terms are not synonymous. Let us briefly examine these in light of community health nursing and the issue of prevention and health promotion.

Case Management

Case management is not to be confused with managed care. Case management can be defined as a variety of approaches to planning, coordinating, and providing care. It is a process of organizing care to attain optimal clinical and fiscally prudent outcomes. Case managers work in acute care settings, public-health nursing settings, in long-term care, and in the insurance industry. Most case managers are brokers of services, i.e., they do not directly provide the care but arrange for it to be done by another party or agency with cost for providing the service as a major factor in selecting the provider.

In some organizations, the case manager is the gatekeeper for care, removing the option of decision making from virtually all providers and transferring it from the patient and family to the payer. This seems to be a veiled effort at rationing care according to resources. Whether case management actually saves money and minimizes unnecessary use of limited services is not yet certain. The role of prevention and health promotion is never mentioned in any of the case management literature despite the fact that this approach to providing health care is gaining in popularity.

Managed Care

In the managed care scheme, the subscriber chooses from a range of providers and settings for the services of managing and coordinating care that will meet his or her needs. It is an arrangement of health care goals, i.e., a grouping of acceptable patients in agency settings and by providers who are using this mechanism for controlling health care costs. Some might wish to describe managed care as a forum for managing benefits, not care, and of rationing care according to what the "manager" deems appropriate in view of who employs that manager and who orchestrates the access to benefits and care considered appropriate for the subscriber. The role of prevention and health promotion are not evident in this approach to health care delivery.

Managed Competition

In managed competition, individuals are placed into groups overseen by a sponsor who negotiates coverage with a fixed panel of physicians and hospitals and who monitors treatment. Health care providers—presumably physicians, HMOs, or hospitals—compete to win contracts from the sponsors and are required to offer high-quality care at attractive prices. A question that arises from this approach is whether there is competition in health care, or just a lot of advertising? Costs of managing care and competition are only now being evaluated, but this direction for delivering care appears to be expensive and has given rise to another category of health worker—who is often a nurse—as manager of benefits. Rather than being methods of providing health care, both managed care and managed competition are vehicles of payment for health care. Again, prevention and health promotion interventions are not mentioned when these approaches to health care delivery are described in the literature.

Managed Public Health Care

The provision and funding of a managed public health-care program with an emphasis on prevention and health promotion is not likely to be considered by payers, but why not think about it? This approach would place prevention in the same league as high technology and acute care but with an interesting twist: Interventions for prevention could be organized for optimal outcomes from a health delivery source chosen by the subscriber. This might well include alternative health providers using herbal or homeopathic products and natural foods as a preventive measure in one's diet, in addition to more traditional approaches to prevention of illnesses.

In a managed public health-care system, the decision as to whether a subscriber could access care would depend on life style and the likelihood that the care would be successful in its outcome. If so, that intervention would be approved. Of course, only selected individuals would be approved in order to predict a cost-effective outcome. If money is made available to pay for services—whether for prevention or treatment of a known disorder—cost would be measured by what is saved rather than what is spent. Typically, prevention has been supported with hard-won public funds. Would managed public health care fall into that continuing pattern, or would it follow the managed care approach where the benefit is managed rather than the care?

In the case management approach, community health nursing visits for prevention and health promotion would require approval from the broker who is the designated manager. In this model, the nurse provider is not given the prerogative of the decision for care but is advised by the broker as to what is acceptable for care and reimbursement. This methodology would be reluctantly accepted by the nurse directed to provide the care for prevention.

Nurses cannot be ignorant about the financing for nursing services. In the past, nurses were either not included in the rate structure or, if included, the services of prevention and health promotion were not regarded as a primary cost center but as a non-reimbursable add-on. This is because, in part, nurses have been careless about defining nursing's role and in describing the action of prevention and health promotion.

In the future, it should be expected that nursing—especially community health nursing in which the scope of practice is so clearly prevention and health promotion—will receive reimbursement for services rendered and documented. Measurement of outcomes will be essential for the positive effect of these services. Changed behavior, improved and more stable health (if a condition exists), and acceptable costs for these services will result.

Potentials for the Future of Community Health Nursing Practice

Identifying the "market share" might be one approach toward considering future potentials for community health nursing. For instance, a community health agency that has a smoking cessation program, sponsored by a for-profit agency and popular, funded, and achieving results, should continue its effective work. For a public-sponsored agency to compete with another similar program would be diverting funds that could go toward a prevention clinic at the local high school or an exercise program for elderly individuals who attend a common meal site. Duplication of prevention and health promotion services must be avoided to save money.

Payment for some public health services might come from a federal income tax check-off similar to that used for the presidential election fund. Such a program would go a long way toward augmenting regularly allocated federal support for programs such as prevention of the maternal/child health problems of malnutrition or abuse, reduction of communicable disease through education, and distribution of information about life styles, helping prevent hypertension, stroke, or cancer.

The federal government, through the Public Health Service, is carrying out its responsibilities by providing leadership and cooperation with state and local health departments, with private and nonprofit provider groups, and with health professionals who provide direct preventive and clinical services, as well as with the people who receive those services ("A Plan to Strengthen" 1991, p. 5). This initiative focuses specifically on prevention and health promotion and identifies strategies and actions for capacity building in the core functions of assessment, policy development, and assurance. It directs research on prevention over the five-year period from January 1991 through January 1996, establishes evaluation measures to document progress and to identify needs for new research, and provides leadership and assistance in upgrading the knowledge and skills of public health workers at the local, state, and national levels.

Excellence in Practice

New opportunities will surface in community health practice and nurses must be front and center in accepting roles of leadership and responsibility. One example is the future development of community nursing centers or organizations to assist in prevention and health promotion services while eventually replacing hospitals as primary providers of health care. These centers will be staffed by nurses and will likely be financially structured on a capitation-fee model within which all health care needs will be provided for the consumer at a specific rate. This model of health care delivery holds much promise and it will be community health nursing that will determine its success.

Education and Service

In the future, we must accept only quality educational opportunities for students that come through institutions that have worked toward excellence and that have rigorous performance standards for all faculty, including the clinical faculty. Should the community nursing agency find that the quality of the educational experience is less than excellent, it should correct this and place the school on notice to improve it. Similarly, schools should not be so desperate for clinical placements that they accept poorly organized and executed clinical services as an experience for the students.

There is a large and growing cohort of students who are in nursing education programs and who never actually receive formal directed education, including the theory and the field practice. Since this is a well-known and specific body of knowledge, how can it be that a nurse is considered proficient in a practice for which there has been no theory and no supervised clinical practice? What other specialty profession would believe that to be an acceptable equivalent? No matter what the educational level of the student might be—and especially with the basic student nurse—there must be a commitment of the community health nursing agency to provide appropriate and essential supervised clinical experiences for optimal preparation of the student nurse.

We must agree on a major approach to the education of community health nurses, at any level of formal learning, that is not exploitive but that is developed with honesty and integrity. No shortcuts in education should be tolerated. Shared expertise between the service agency and the educational institution should increase: sharing resources will enhance the goals of both service and education. Service agencies should plan with college faculty to provide all students who come the very best and the most rigorous clinical experience available.

Competent work in the community includes care for all age groups, all cultures, and for all clinical needs, including prevention, and acute and chronic interventions. This mandate is not for everyone. We must be certain that only the best and the most competent are involved.

Excellence in practice requires moral leadership, too. Nurses will have to demonstrate exquisite clinical practice skills and a commitment to basic values, to earning the trust of patients and colleagues, and to the work ethic of fairness.

Conclusion

In community health nursing, the potentials for prevention and health promotion as an integral part of future health care delivery are promising. Nurses must cultivate habits that lead to new ideas, an expansion of the scope of nursing practice, and creative methods of providing and paying for all of the essential prevention and health promotion services rendered by nurses. Nurses have the capacity to do it and are limited only if their reach exceeds their grasp.

References

American Public Health Association. 1991. *Healthy communities 2000: Model standards* (3rd ed.). Washington, DC: Author.
Institute of Medicine. 1988. *The future of public health.* Washington, DC: National Academy Press.
Office of Assistant Secretary for Health and Surgeon General. 1979. *Healthy people. The Surgeon General's report on health promotion and disease prevention.* Washington, DC: U.S. Government Printing Office.
A plan to strengthen public health in the United States. Public Health Reports. 1991. Vol. 106. Supplement #1.
Castro, J. "Condition: Critical." *Time.* November 25, 1991: 32–42.
U.S. Department of Health and Human Services, U.S. Public Health Service. 1990. *Healthy people 2000: National health promotion and disease prevention objectives.* Washington, DC, U.S. Government Printing Office.
World Health Organization. 1977. *Global strategy for health for all by the year 2000.* Geneva, Switzerland: Author.

ABOUT THE AUTHORS

Theresa Apriceno-Tesoro, M.S.N., R.N., C.S., P.N.P. is a lecturer/clinical specialist in the Primary Care Graduate Program at the University of Pennsylvania School of Nursing, Philadelphia, Pennsylvania.

Kathleen B. Blomquist, Ph.D., R.N., M.S.N., M.P.H. is an assistant research professor at the Sanders-Brown Center on Aging at the University of Kentucky in Lexington.

John Fehir, Ph.D., R.N., C. is an evaluation consultant for the W.K. Kellogg-funded De Madres a Madres program in Houston, Texas.

Beverly C. Flynn, Ph.D., R.N., F.A.A.N. is a professor at the Indiana University School of Nursing, Department of Community Health Nursing in Indianapolis. She is also the Director of the Institute of Action Research for Community Health; Head of the World Health Organization Collaborating Center in Healthy Cities; and Director, CITYNET Healthy Cities.

Jean Goeppinger, Ph.D., R.N., F.A.A.N. is Professor and Chair, Department of Community and Mental Health Nursing, School of Nursing, the University of North Carolina, Chapel Hill.

Janet Heinrich, Ph.D., R.N., F.A.A.N. is the Executive Director of the American Academy of Nursing, Washington, DC. She was the former director of the Division of Extramural Programs, National Center for Nursing Research, National Institutes of Health, in Bethesda, Maryland.

O. Marie Henry, D.N.Sc., R.N., F.A.A.N. recently retired from her position as Deputy Surgeon General, Public Health Service, U.S. Department of Health and Human Services.

Ada Sue Hinshaw, Ph.D., R.N., F.A.A.N. is Director of the National Institute of Nursing Research at the National Institutes of Health.

Constance A. Holleran, M.S.N., R.N., F.A.A.N. is the Executive Director of the International Council of Nurses in Geneva, Switzerland.

Judith B. Igoe, M.S., R.N., F.A.A.N. is an associate professor and Director, School Health Programs at the University of Colorado Health Sciences Center in Denver.

Ruth N. Knollmueller, Ph.D., R.N. is on the faculty at the University of Connecticut School of Nursing, Storrs, and former assistant director of the Waterbury, Connecticut branch of Visiting Nurse And Home Care, Inc. She is also the coauthor of the *Handbook of Community and Home Health Nursing: Tools in Assessment, Intervention and Education.*

Carol Macnee, Ph.D., R.N. is an Associate Professor of Family-Community Nursing at East Tennessee State University in Johnson City, Tennessee.

Judith McFarlane, Dr.P.H., R.N., F.A.A.N. is a professor of community health nursing at the College of Nursing, Texas Woman's University in Houston. She is also the Director of De Madres a Madres, and principal investigator of the Centers for Disease Control grant, Abuse during Pregnancy.

Ann L. O'Sullivan, Ph.D., R.N., F.A.A.N. is an associate professor at the University of Pennsylvania School of Nursing, and a pediatric nurse practitioner at The Children's Hospital of Philadelphia.

Carol Patwari, B.S.N., R.N. is the Communicable Disease Program Coordinator at the Harris County Health Department in Houston, Texas.

Joanne W. Rains, D.N.Sc., R.N. is an assistant professor at the Indiana University School of Nursing, Department of Community Health Nursing. She is also Fellow, Institute of Action Research for Community Health, and Fellow, World Health Organization Collaborating Center in Healthy Cities.

Marla E. Salmon, Sc.D., R.N., F.A.A.N. is Director of the Division of Nursing of the Bureau of Health Professions, Health Resources and Services Administration, Public Health Service, U.S. Department of Health and Human Services, in Rockville, Maryland.

Susan J. Simmons, Ph.D., R.N. is Senior Policy Analyst with the Office on Women's Health, Public Health Service, U.S. Department of Health and Human Services in Washington, DC.

Gloria R. Smith, Ph.D., R.N., F.A.A.N. is Program Director and Coordinator of Health Programming at the W.K. Kellogg Foundation in Battle Creek, Michigan.

Rachel E. Spector, Ph.D., R.N., C.T.N. is an associate professor at the Boston College School of Nursing in Chestnut Hill, Massachusetts. She is also the elected Chair of the Needham, Massachusetts Board of Health, and is the author of *Cultural Diversity in Health and Illness*.

Ruby Wesley, Ph.D., R.N. is the Director of Nursing Practice at The Rehabilitation Institute of Michigan and an Assistant Professor of Nursing at Wayne State University College of Nursing, both in Detroit, Michigan.

Carolyn A. Williams, Ph.D., R.N., F.A.A.N. is Dean and Professor of Community Health Nursing at the College of Nursing, University of Kentucky in Lexington.

DATE DUE

JUN 2 6 2003

GAYLORD   PRINTED IN U.S.A.

Demco, Inc. 38-293